HEALING —THE— MIND AND BODY

VOLUME 1

SECOND EDITION

UNLOCK THE SECRET TRUTHS ABOUT THE MIND-BODY CONNECTION TO ACHIEVE OPTIMAL MIND-BODY HARMONY AND HEALTH

PAUL D. CORONA, M.D.

Edited by
Tom Herron &
Chuck Smith, Jr.

The Corona Protocol

Foreword by
Chuck Smith, Jr.

Healing the Mind and Body: The Trilogy
Volume 1, Second Edition by Paul D. Corona, M.D.

Hardcover: 979-8-9896000-4-5
Paperback: 979-8-9896000-3-8
eBook: 979-8-9896000-5-2
LCCN: 2025923071

Published by: The Corona Protocol,
30011 Ivy Glenn Dr., Suite 101, Laguna Niguel, CA 92677
www.drpaulcoronamd.com

Edited by Tom Herron & Chuck Smith, Jr.
Foreword by Chuck Smith, Jr.
Illustrations by Christi Koop, K-2 Graphix
Cover design by Jaime Simon
Second Edition Interior Design by Karen Corriente

Second Edition Printing, 2026

Library of Congress Cataloguing-in-Publication
Corona, M.D., Paul D.
Healing the Mind and Body: Volume 1, Second Edition
Paul D. Corona, M.D. p.428

AUTHOR'S NOTE

The subject of neurochemical imbalances is a complex field of study. I have therefore made every effort to present the subject so it can be easily understood by all who wish to learn more about the mind-body connection and the integral role it plays in one's life. Nevertheless, there are times when explaining how the mind and body interact requires the introduction of peripheral material. Should you find any of this material too technical, simply skip ahead to a section where you feel more comfortable. I am confident that as you refer to this book to seek answers to your questions you will become increasingly more knowledgeable about this subject and come to understand not just some, but all of the contents.

DISCLAIMER

The information in this book, *Healing the Mind and Body 1,* is intended to serve strictly as reference material. It is not to be construed as medical or professional advice. The information contained herein is intended to provide you with the tools to make informed decisions about your health and lifestyle. It should not be used as a substitute for any form of treatment that has been prescribed or recommended by your doctor.

The author and publisher expressly disclaim any and all responsibility for any adverse effects resulting from the use of the suggestions or information herein. This book is offered as current information obtained from the author's practical experience about neurochemical imbalances and their effect on one's health. Furthermore, the information in this book is provided for your own education and enjoyment. If you suspect you have a neurochemical imbalance, it is imperative that you seek medical attention from a qualified healthcare professional. Under no circumstances should you attempt to implement any of the ideas contained herein without the care and guidance of such a professional.

TABLE OF CONTENTS

SECTION II – **The Technology of Moods**

SECTION III – **The State of Medicine and How it is Affecting the Mind and Body of The Patient**

Dedication

The Corona Protocol is dedicated to my wife, Denise, and my two children, Logan and Baylee. They have put up with my endless hours of work over the years and have been very patient and understanding, at least most of the time. They are the most important parts of my life, and I will try my best to make it up to them. It has been difficult to balance writing this book with a busy clinical practice while trying to maintain a healthy home life, but it has been fun trying.

My beautiful wife, Denise, is truly my soul mate. She is as beautiful on the inside as she is on the outside, and when I look into her eyes I understand the true meaning of love, art and the joy of the life that I share with her.

My children are the jewels of my life, and I experience no greater joy than when I am with them. I am proud of their accomplishments and I pray for all the best for them in the future.

I also dedicate The Corona Protocol to my father, Arthur. He has been my role model, advisor, confidant and best friend. He taught me the importance of having a passion for what one does. He has been immeasurably supportive over the years in many different ways, and I thank him for that. I am looking forward to spending more time with him in the future. I could not ask for a better father.

I dedicate this body of work to God and thank Him for giving me the strength to write it. I have felt very much in communion with God during the writing of this book. It has been an incredible journey of discovery, and I have very much enjoyed traveling it. I pray that The Corona Protocol makes a difference in your life by providing you the hope that you desire and a fuller sense of well-being and happiness, and I hope you are able to realize your dreams.

FOREWORD

Mention *Fibromyalgia* to ten people in the healthcare industry and seven of them will roll their eyes. Why do people, even professionals, sometimes react this way to conditions like *Fibromyalgia, Chronic Fatigue Syndrome, Irritable Bowel Syndrome, TMJ Syndrome,* and other stress-related illnesses, as if someone had used the word *hypochondriac?* For one simple reason: The actual condition that manifests as *Fibromyalgia* cannot be located in the human body with any of the conventional diagnostic tools, such as x-rays or blood tests. If someone suffers from a disorder that seems to be purely stress-related, it is assumed that the person is weak, neurotic, a complainer, and somehow responsible for their illness.

Of course this thinking is inconsistent and illogical. For example, we would not say that a man who had a stress-related heart attack brought it on himself if we found out he was suffering from a heart disease. If a woman's diabetes flares up when she is under stress, we do not hold her responsible. Most of us are well aware of the ways we are affected by stress and how it amplifies irritability, sensitivity to noise and confusion (which we can normally tolerate), and the unpleasant way certain people affect us.

Some people assume that doctors tell annoying patients they have a condition with an exotic name like *"Fibromyalgia,"* so they will respond to a placebo. Those same people think that the condition is "all in his head," and worry that giving it a label will make him feel that all his whining is justified. They can go home from the doctor's office and tell their families, "See! There really is something wrong with me!"

There are doctors and their staff who dread seeing these patients come through the door, because they know that no matter what treatment they prescribe, those folks are simply not going to get better. Fibromyalgia is not all in a person's head, although what is happening in their bodies is sensitive to chemical conditions in their brain and central nervous system. The disorders that have so far evaded detection are destroying millions upon millions of human lives.

Dr. Corona understands the real pain, fatigue, and despair people experience when they are plagued by conditions that others in the medical community have yet to take seriously. His wisdom is revealed in the fact that he knows the weakness and despair of chronic fatigue syndrome, the hopelessness of depression, and the agony of the unrelenting pain of TMJ are all real conditions—the pain is real, the inability to fight off despair is real, the collapse of the body's immune system is real, and a host of other symptoms are also real. Dr. Corona's compassion is shown in the fact that he lets these patients know, "You have an extremely painful and unpredictable condition that is real, and that is not your fault. You are suffering, but you haven't done anything to bring this on yourself and you do not deserve it. Nor is there anything you can do through willpower or positive thinking that will make it go away." Dr. Corona's genius is the discovery of cures for these patients through a painstaking process of treating them one at a time and evaluating their individual physical, neurological, mental, and environmental situations and the specific targeting of medications to resolve the source of the problem and not merely relieve symptoms.

Can Dr. Corona work miracles? No. Do the medications he prescribes work miracles? No. The results he achieves have a scientific and rational basis. To the person who has been depressed, the emotional change, positive outlook, and even the presence of hope feels like a miracle. The same is true of people who suffer from bipolar disorder or chronic fatigue disorder. Prior to meeting Dr. Corona, these people believed that healing and the recovery of the happiness of their youth was impossible. After their treatment, the dark thoughts, that were once so familiar, become alien to them and hope becomes their new state of mind.

I would hope that this book moves rapidly into every corner of our society and is widely read, because it has the potential to ease suffering, point the way to healing, give people a real chance at life, and mend broken families. I am grateful that I met Dr. Paul when I did, and that he won my confidence. I am a different person today due to his willingness to walk with me through my own mental quagmire and into a much better place. In the same way that I have referred dozens of patients to his office, I now recommend Dr. Paul to you. The education you will receive is worth your time. The goal of this book is to help you create the healthiest, happiest life possible, and the subject is you and whatever might be holding you back.

Chuck Smith, Jr.
Author of *There Is A Season* and *Frequently Avoided Questions*.

About the Editor: Chuck Smith, Jr., is an author and Soul-Care provider at *Reflexion–a Spiritual Community* (http://www.reflexionsc.net/). Having lived with depression for nearly 40 years, he has an avid interest in recent breakthroughs in neuropsychology regarding neuroplasticity, the treatment of mood disorders, and how positive changes can be affected by the Central Nervous System through spiritual disciplines such as prayer and meditation. His books include *There Is A Season, Frequently Avoided Questions, Epiphany: Discover the Delight of God's Word* and *Memoirs of Grace* (the biography of his father Chuck Smith, founder of Calvary Chapel). He lives in Dana Point, California with his wife Barbara Smith, PT, who is also his best friend.

Introduction

The idea of first writing The Corona Protocol came to me while I was sitting in Communion at church. At first it was a passing thought I assumed I could ignore. Steadily the many life-enhancing insights I had discovered in my medical practice crowded into my brain, and I realized it was my responsibility to publish this information for the benefit of others. The decision was clinched later that evening in a local Chinese restaurant as I discussed the book idea with my wife, Denise, and broke open a fortune cookie to find, "An important decision will take place today." So, after the children were tucked into their beds, I immediately went to my desk and began writing.

The inspiration that drove me was a fundamental premise: Mood disorders are caused by neurochemical imbalances that prevent the brain and body from functioning properly. Hours passed like minutes, words turned into sentences, sentences turned into paragraphs as I filled page after page. My scribbled thoughts began to take a definitive shape, and as they did, I came to a stunning realization. During the course of practicing medicine for over twenty-five years, I had made a discovery that I had not read about in any of the journals or heard from anyone else in the medical community, and one that I felt obligated to share with the world.

When registering for pre-med courses I was not planning the future in which I would be treating mood disorders. Like most of my colleagues in the medical profession, my deepest desire was to work at improving the health of my patients by addressing physical complaints with organic causes such as illness, injury, organ malfunction and so on. What I discovered in years of Family Practice is that more than half, more likely three quarters, of my patients' complaints were either caused or exacerbated by "emotional" issues (I place quotation marks around emotional, because emotions arise from neurological activity in the brain). Moreover, the number of patients or family members who struggled from increased stress, worry or fear due to physical complaints and how well they were prepared to respond to it logistically, financially, etcetera, rose to a figure closer to one hundred percent.

Once I turned my attention to the underlying neurological factors in health care, I witnessed remarkable changes in my patients who were frankly sick and tired of being sick and tired. Even those with an illness for which modern medicine had no known cure (such as Fibromyalgia, Irritable Bowel Syndrome, Chronic Fatigue Syndrome, any recurrent and chronic pain, or whichever chronic and recurring problems whose etiology is unknown), showed marked improvement in their attitudes in dealing with both their ailments and with life in general. At the same time, their complaints diminished and in many cases were fully resolved.

I assured them that these neurological conditions were not their fault, and that there was hope even when things seemed hopeless.

No other option presented itself to me other than an aggressive pursuit towards the best treatment for these primary threats to human health and happiness. The further I went, the more I learned that more of my patients benefited from my research and clinical practice. In the process of moving forward I have come to appreciate minor failures and setbacks, learning from them as much (sometimes more) as from my successes. The more I did it and practiced I was getting more and more hits and less and less misses, since practice makes perfect. (It's called a medical practice because we just keep practicing until we get it right.) Eventually, all of these factors evolved into a rational trial-and-error algorithmic approach to treating mood disorders: The Corona Protocol.

The Corona Protocol differs from the fairly standard procedure of prescribing one of the known anti-anxiety medications to a patient whose complaints and symptoms indicate anxiety. There are several problems with this approach, including the fact that innumerable chemical variations differentiate one patient from another, determining what works for each individual and also what sort of side effects the medication may produce and whether they can be tolerated. When doctors prescribe a medication to a patient that they do not know well enough and whose case they have not thoroughly researched, they are rolling the dice hoping for a favorable outcome. When one medication proves to be ineffective, the prescribing physician may increase the dose and give it more time or move on to something else, leaving many patients wondering whether they are viewed as lab rats.

At its core, The Corona Protocol is an evidence-based detailed approach to health care. There are clear and proven reasons for every step taken in treating mood disorders, down to the finest details. Not only is the family history more extensive than what Family Physicians typically require, The Corona Protocol does not allow the patient's doctor to skim over it, but rather to read and research it carefully, paying close attention to detail. The family history in developing a differential diagnosis for treating mood disorders is indispensable because indications of genetic predispositions are invaluable for determining the likely neurochemical components in need of attention. No shortcuts can be taken in this regard. The better a doctor understands what is happening in the patient's neurochemistry, the more precisely he or she is able to choose from the host of excellent available psychotropic medications, which lead to truly amazing results when they are mixed together correctly in order to optimize the results emotionally and physically.

The same sort of "close look" approach is applied to the patient's personal history and specific symptoms. In so much as mood disorders tend to overlap—for example, the anxious person may experience bouts of depression and the depressive patient may be tortured by repetitive and anxious thoughts—the doctor must be well-informed to decide how to best approach the treatment based on the history and symptoms. Stories of unhealthy home environments, abuse, trauma, at-risk adolescent behavior and so on, which enables the physician to clarify the diagnosis. Once again, the more accurate the information and thus diagnosis, the more sensible the choices made in determining which of the incredible variety of medications we are able to prescribe.

An initial goal of The Corona Protocol is that the first medication prescribed is also the best and most effective for that individual. Then we need to find the best augmenting agents in order to create the perfect mix for that person. This goal is neither easily or consistently attained, but having a rational process consistently produces better results than shooting in the dark.

Malcolm Gladwell in his book *Blink* discusses the fascinating topic of Thin-slicing, which I will discuss later. He also explains that if a person's work consists of 10,000 hours of experience, that person is an expert in that craft. I have spent more than 50,000 hours practicing this method, and I'm still having fun learning how to do it better and better as I continue (and it's fun to see the results and witness a life changed for the better). I'm excited to share my method with you, and I hope it helps you and your patients.

Throughout my practice I have always listened intently to my patients. After all, they know their symptoms better than anyone else. I have always returned their phone calls, listened to their complaints, and asked them for feedback after providing treatment or prescribing medications and noting the detailed responses to each intervention. I have thoroughly enjoyed learning medicine from them and their individual responses to treatment and discovering the physical and psychological reasons why some respond better than others. The more I spoke with them, the more my education in human health and well-being deepened. Eventually, this subject became the major theme of my practice. I have now seen literally tens of thousands of patients, and as a result, I have made a discovery that is both intriguing and absolutely fascinating. What is this amazing discovery? Simply, the mind-body connection is the single most important topic in medicine today, by far. Sadly, however, it is also the "missing link" of medicine.

The Discovery of the Missing Link

The term missing link is used in science to indicate a jump from one stage of development to another without evidence for transitional stages in-between. The missing link in medicine and psychology has to do with how we get from brain (or neural) states to mood disorders like depression and obsessive-compulsive disorder. In other words, what connects the brain and its body to the mind, the self that we personalize when we say, "I'm feeling really down today."

In this book you will learn the connection between the neural activity in your brain and how you feel emotionally. You will also find a practical guide to recognizing and treating mood disorders and a variety of physical symptoms that can be traced back to chemical imbalances in the nervous system.

Specialists in the field of medicine and psychology learn how neurochemical imbalances are responsible for a host of patient complaints that have not been resolved because of inadequate diagnoses—in other words, people in our professions do not usually look for neurochemical causes of many mental and physical symptoms. Once these issues are clearly understood, the professional can proceed with proper treatment or provide their patients with an appropriate referral, leaving them with more time to deal with the problems within the scope of their training. Psychologists, in particular, will find this helpful in understanding when medications may be appropriate and how they can optimize each patient's treatment with a combination of medications and psychotherapy.

Proper recognition and treatment could also prevent unnecessary work-ups and expenditures, saving individuals and the healthcare system a lot of money and resources that could be better spent and used elsewhere. Through greater cooperation in the healthcare industry we will see an increase in the rate of patient improvement. I have always enjoyed the team approach in my practice whenever given the opportunity to work with other doctors, counselors, and religious leaders.

Medical students, Residents and Fellows will find The Corona Protocol invaluable because it contains "how to" instructions regarding patient care that they were not taught in medical schools or specialty training, but are crucial for an effective general or specialized practice. Hopefully they can develop skills in excellence before they have already been locked into bad habits that can be difficult to break. I can assure you that what you will read in the following pages is the most important subject that doctors deal with in the office on a daily basis. Given the fact that medicine is constantly evolving, it is important that we keep up with medical advances and not get stuck in our ways, but rather be open to new treatment possibilities. Fortunately for the human race, new insights into disease, genetics, medicine, and so on, are being reported every week, which means we will always be learning better ways of serving those who come to us for help.

Certainly not least, and in many cases even more so, patients will find The Corona Protocol of enormous value. You are going to be amazed at the way your mind and body work together at times, and work apart at other times, and how this mind-body interaction affects your health in normal and abnormal ways. Equipped with this information, you will have a better understanding of your physicians' goals in treating you and therefore be able to cooperate with them for better results.

FOUNDATIONAL ASSUMPTIONS AND APPLICATIONS

To make the adjustment to better health care, we all must first acknowledge that mood disorders are most commonly rooted in genetics, and that when they occur, they are not the patient's fault. We must also realize that the patient's complaints are real, the problems underlying their symptoms are real, and the medical solutions to these problems are real. Once patients are reassured that the doctor takes them seriously, has knowledge of their condition and is certain that it can be relieved, if not cured, they will have less fear, hesitancy and resistance to their neurochemical imbalances being corrected. This cooperation is a tremendous aid toward healing because addressing these issues as early as possible and treating them aggressively delivers the best results.

Patients and doctors frequently collude to treat a condition with a "band-aid" (a "quick-fix medication" that only treats symptoms rather than prevents them). We make these unwritten agreements when we suspect that the patient's problem is hypochondria, the potential treatments are too risky, painful, or expensive to be acceptable, or we are baffled by the symptoms and honestly do not know how to treat them. We can, however, learn to do better than hide deeper conditions with superficial solutions. Patients can learn ways to take responsibility for, and manage, their own health through prevention, early detection, and full cooperation with their physicians. The patients' greater involvement in their health care means that doctors will need to spend less time trying to convince them of the importance of the prescribed treatment.

My primary resource for the breakthrough information in The Corona Protocol comes from the observations and education acquired through many years of a very busy practice. The benefits to be gained from what you will learn here include:

- Practical tips and "pearls" for doctors who, through their daily practice, want to make a difference.
- A guide for patients who want the truth about mood disorders, how to work with doctors, and how to obtain the best treatment results.
- A baseline understanding in order to make quick and sound decisions for addressing mood disorders. You will see that getting treatment and positive results as quickly as possible is necessary for people suffering from mood disorders.

- Information about the human brain, what is necessary for it to function properly, and how to assist it when there is a malfunction in one or more of its operations.

- The potential to save countless lives and dramatically improve the quality of life for many others.

- Addressing issues in our society that are of serious concern to many of us, such as normalizing aberrant behavior and reducing healthcare expenditures.

Welcome to the cutting-edge of medicine. The recognition and treatment of neurochemical imbalances in the nervous system, is transforming the world of medicine, making it possible for everyone to realize the physical, emotional, relational, and spiritual benefits of the improved balance between the mind and body, functioning as they were designed to function. Most importantly, the net result of exploring this exciting and fascinating topic are the positive changes you will experience as you begin to feel and respond to life the way it was meant to be enjoyed.

ABOUT THE AUTHOR

Paul Daniel Corona was born and raised in Southern California, specifically in the South Bay area of Los Angeles County. He attended the University of Southern California from 1980-1984, where he received a BS degree in Biology/Premed. He then received his M.D. degree from New York Medical College in 1989, and then completed a Family Practice Residency program from 1989 to 1992 at California Medical Center in Los Angeles, and became Board Certified in the specialty of Family Medicine. He and his wife Denise then moved to their current home in south Orange County in 1993, where they have remained and have raised their children, Logan and Baylee.

Dr. Corona has enjoyed practicing the full spectrum of Family Medicine for over 30 years, but had been particularly interested early on in how stress and other emotional symptoms affected the physical body. His early interests became a passion over the years as he became more and more fascinated with what he was seeing and learning, and how common it is once recognized and what an impact treating this had on his patients' lives.

He has treated tens of thousands of patients for neurochemical imbalances over more than 30 years of a very busy clinical practice. For more than a decade and a half, he has devoted his full practice to the recognition and treatment of neurochemical imbalances, and has dedicated the rest of his career to patient care and teaching patients and doctors alike the emotional and physical benefits of this revolutionary medical solution that can change your life for the better and help you to achieve your goals and realize your dreams.

HEALING
— THE —
MIND AND BODY
VOLUME 1
SECOND EDITION

— SECTION I —

- THE WOW
- MYTHS AND MISCONCEPTIONS

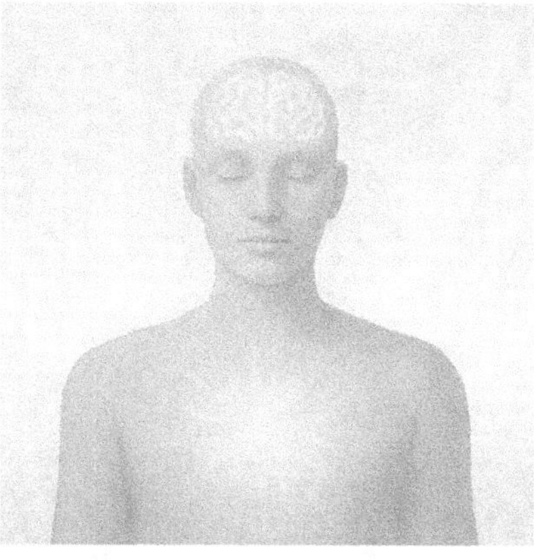

PAUL D. CORONA, M.D.

CHAPTER ONE

THE WOW

What is the WOW of emotional health? Quite simply it is the Wonder of Optimal Well-being, and it is available to everyone.

The WOW is for everyone, even for those who have experienced years of frustration because of anxiety or depression, or for those who have suffered from chronic fatigue or other physical aches and pains. The WOW is readily available for all who are sick and tired of being sick and tired. The hope lies in the underrated and often misunderstood chemistry of the brain, where even a slight adjustment can make the difference between enjoying the WOW or suffering the WOE (Whacked Out Equilibrium).

The tools for making those adjustments are now in the hands of physicians, with improvements being added every year. Working with you, a qualified healthcare provider can diagnose and address emotional and physical complaints that are caused by chemical imbalances.[1] You will definitely know when the right adjustments have been made, because you will experience a new sense of well being, a positive attitude, and enjoyment of life. In fact, many patients have described the difference as a radical transformation that has turned them into a new person. Some patients have said to me, "So Dr. Paul, if this is what *normal* feels like, I love it!"

This book in your hands is a powerful tool that will explain the full potential of the WOW and guide you to it. In the pages that follow, you will learn about the chemical and biological functions that are necessary to feel good, both mentally and emotionally. My goal for you is the same as I have always had for every patient of mine: To help you have the best possible experience of life, enjoying it rather than merely surviving. If you already feel wonderful in life and have no need for this book, then think of a friend or family member who can benefit from finding out why happiness has always eluded them. Sharing what you find here could even save someone's life.

1 Later we will explore the radical chemical changes that occur with growth, significant physical events—such as childbirth or surgery—and aging. These changes are normal functions of the human body, but can sometimes result in unhealthy and undesired alterations in neurological functions.

THE HEART OF THE MATTER (AND MATTERS OF THE HEART)

Many people in North America and all over the world are suffering needlessly. Some of these people have been led to believe their condition is chronic and they will have to suffer with it for the rest of their lives. The truth is, in the majority of cases the problem is treatable, but undiagnosed, because their physicians have failed to determine the cause of their symptoms.

There is a common prejudice that is characteristic of both patients and doctors and it works against healing and wellness: They refuse to believe what they cannot see. We *know* the body has a circulatory system, endocrine system, organs, and tissue that can be examined in x-rays, MRIs, scans, and in some cases "exploratory surgery." The functions of the central nervous system, which is the most crucial system of all, are mostly hidden from our best diagnostic technology. That does not mean, however, that diagnosing neural problems is impossible, but that we must go about it in a different manner, one that does not require a direct line of sight.

Many patients have a difficult time with an "invisible" cause for their symptoms, and since they know they are not crazy or imagining their pain, they tend to resist, at first, the idea that I cannot show them what is going wrong inside their body. To help ease them into this new way of understanding the diagnosis of chemical imbalances, I may use a "light switch" analogy. I ask them to think about the wires in the wall that connect the wall switch to the light. If a wire inside the wall has for some reason a kink in it, then electricity cannot flow through it efficiently and this causes the light to go on and off. How do we know the wire is broken if we cannot see it? Well, we flip the switch. If the light does not go on, we check the bulb and all the visible parts. If we cannot find a problem with any of the fixtures or places where the wire connects, then it is more certain than a guess that there is a break in the wire somewhere that is not visible to us.

The same reasoning holds for the central nervous system. In this case though we are dealing with chemicals as well as electricity. Neurochemical imbalances are both a plumbing and electrical malfunction. X-rays and lab tests will not tell us what serotonin or dopamine are doing within the synaptic gaps between neurons (do not get nervous, because you will easily understand these terms later on when I explain them to you), but we know what is supposed to happen when they function properly. If symptoms indicate they are not doing what they are supposed to do, and we have ruled out any visible or obvious factors, then we can be quite certain that they need some adjusting.

Doctors and patients feel a sense of relief when a name can be tagged onto the patient's complaint with a corresponding knowledge of a known cure. When doctors scratch their heads every time they look at x-rays or test results and tell the patient, "We simply cannot find anything wrong with you," the poor sufferer often collapses into a cycle of worsening symptoms. The reason their condition becomes worse is because not knowing the cause of their condition fills them with a sense of powerlessness and lack of control that even their doctors are unable to address. Feeling hopeless is the worst feeling of all. The extra stress that weighs on patients takes an even greater toll on their body, and especially their immune system, which intensifies their symptoms. We can break this cycle.

Every doctor has experienced the frustration of having patients who do not improve no matter what medication, surgery, or therapy has been applied to their condition. These are the patients that make repeated office visits to complain of vague illnesses or pains that, medically speaking, do not make sense. Blanket terms have been adopted to give patients the impression that the doctor actually knows the physical cause of their symptoms, including fibromyalgia, irritable bowel syndrome (IBS), chronic fatigue syndrome (CFS), chronic insomnia, or chronic pain syndrome (CPS). Doctors use these terms when they cannot isolate a specific cause for the symptoms. We may feel we are helping our patients by giving them a name for their condition, but our labels are worthless if they do not help us correct the problem.

Through years of practice, ongoing research, and close observation of my patients, I have discovered that many of the strange conditions that defy diagnosis can be easily and effectively treated using

The Corona Protocol, which yields surprisingly positive results. We begin, of course, with the body itself, examining the health and function of organs, glands, tissues, muscles, and bones. If we do not find a clear cause of the persistent symptoms, I suggest we look elsewhere, focusing on what is happening (or not happening) in the extremely small gaps between neurons in the brain and throughout the nervous system.

Naturally we are more comfortable with a condition that is visible on an x-ray or results of lab tests, because we can see a tangible cause, which helps us determine how it can best be resolved. At present, no test is available to doctors that can show them what is happening to the neurotransmitters in the brain. The breakthrough, however, is knowing that if we understand the effects of neurotransmitters when they function properly, then we are able to make educated assumptions about how to go about balancing those chemicals based on the patient's symptoms. For now, the symptom-based approach is a tested and reliable way to diagnose a patient's condition, which I refer to as *the patient-centered* approach to health care. Sadly, as I will explain in more detail later, there are too few doctors who take the time to really listen to their patients or get all the information they need from them to make this method work.

YOUR NEW HORIZON

If you feel like I have been moving too fast through the complex issues of mood disorders and medical terminology, do not worry. The further you read, the more this whole field of health care will be explained until you are comfortable with your knowledge of causes and cures. Then the light will start going on for you—the light of understanding and more importantly the light of hope. For anyone who has suffered from the subtle imbalance of neurochemicals, this book offers the hope of:

- Improved energy and metabolism
- Improved mood
- Greater concentration
- Enhanced memory
- Increased motivation
- Decrease in somatic/pain symptoms
- Better sexual functioning
- Feeling themselves again/feeling normal
- Increased energy
- Improved metabolism
- Improved mood/happier
- Better sleep quality
- Reduced stress/able to handle stress better

As with many other patients before you, after receiving the treatment I describe here, you will likely experience an overall feeling of happiness that will be brand new to you. You will also discover a *ripple effect* as your improved mental and physical condition moves outward, changing and improving your relationships with your family and friends.

The Science and the Art

Doctors have the foundation to begin the effective treatment of mood disorders. Western medicine currently stands in the best position to provide *real, holistic,* and *preventative* treatments of the debilitating emotional conditions that have so many people feeling deeply discouraged or even hopeless about their lives. What we have learned about the brain in recent decades has resulted in major advances in our understanding of how to correct its malfunctions. New breakthroughs in this exciting field are occurring exponentially, and our knowledge grows accordingly. We can now assist the brain in its relentless work of regulating our bodies and moods. With some fundamental training, primary care can take a more active role in recognizing and treating mood disorders. This is the science of the WOW.

In addition to being a science, there is an art to the WOW. From the doctor's point of view, working with the medications that are effective in relieving mood disorders is a creative type of *fun*, because following our educated instincts and collaborating with our patients, we are rewarded with the pleasure of seeing the joy patients have when treatment produces satisfying results.

The Doctor-Patient Partnership

Doctors and patients who are committed to getting the best possible results from mood-altering

(I prefer mood-normalizing) medications are those who develop and maintain a balanced partnership.[2] Patients need to learn something about their brains, bodies, and the interplay between them. They also need to provide their doctors with a list of symptoms, a family history, and a personal history. Doctors, on the other hand, need to connect with each patient and appreciate his or her unique condition, symptoms, response to medicines, and history. Together we are pursuing the ultimate goal of pure happiness and joy, or as close as we can get. Reaching this goal requires us to respect each other, work together, and keep our communication as current and complete as possible. The reward is well worth the effort.

The Book in Brief

The following is an outline of the bedrock principles that led to my methods and protocol regarding my approach to the use of mood-normalizing medications. The information and guidelines in the chapters that follow are built upon these principles regarding mood disorders and their treatment.

1. The interplay between the brain and body is a crucial factor in mood disorders. Every feeling and emotion we experience is connected to,

2 I prefer the term mood-normalizing over mood-altering. For the remainder of the book I will refer to mood-normalizing medications, because we administer them merely to assist the brain to do what it is supposed to do when functioning normally.

and dependent on, a corresponding activity within the brain. Mood disorders are caused by neurochemical imbalances that prevent the brain and the rest of the nervous system from functioning properly.

2. Neurochemical imbalances are the most underdiagnosed and under-treated medical problems in the world today, by far. Many people, at least countless millions to billions, are suffering needlessly simply because neurochemical imbalances are far more common than most people realize. The resolution of this condition already exists in the human body, but it needs assistance to function properly.

3. A number of factors in our society today are causing an increase in mood disorders. These include stress, poor diet, improper or lack of exercise, dysfunctional relationships, irregular sleep, and lack of a spiritual center. These, and many other factors, can be related to mood disorders in a self-perpetuating cycle of cause and effect.

4. Many different events can result in neurochemical imbalances. The most commonly seen problem has to do with genetics. The stronger the genetic factors, the more likely it is that a person will develop a neurochemical imbalance at some point in her or his life. Of course, it

goes without saying that people are not responsible for the genes they inherit, yet many people feel a deep sense of guilt that they cannot be happy—this is especially true of some religious people who think that if they had more faith and hope they would not be depressed. No one is to blame for brain chemistry that is not under his or her control. All we need to do is accept the fact that we have the condition and then deal with it head-on.

5. Incidences of neurochemical imbalances are not necessarily increasing, although an increasing number of such cases are turning up every year, since it is being recognized more often. Thankfully, doctors can now be better informed and trained to recognize and diagnose the cause of problems that seemed untreatable only twenty years ago.

6. Medications that are currently available for treating mood disorders are remarkably effective. Through clinical practice, doctors have discovered that antidepressants also work well on other conditions. These include anxiety disorders and chronic pain disorders. There are many more *off-label* uses for these medications than there are *on-label* uses. *Off-label* means using medications in ways that they weren't originally intended to be used, which often leads to many other uses and exciting treatment

possibilities. In my opinion, *off-label* means *cutting edge*. This will be explained more later on.

The careful and monitored application of these medications guarantees that most patients can enjoy happier and healthier lives.

7. Anyone can suffer from a chemical imbalance. The onset can occur at any age, even if the patient has enjoyed sixty years of normal emotional health.

8. By and large, the international medical community does not recognize the importance of the medications that are now available for treating disorders that are caused by neurochemical imbalances. To date, there are no standardized procedures for prescribing mood-normalizing medications, and the conventional wisdom of increasing doses of the same medication until a patient reports improvement is wrong for reasons that will become clear later in the book. I will reveal to you why The Corona Protocol is so much more of an efficient, effective and ultimately rational solution than what has been available up until now.

9. Every person and situation is unique and requires specialized treatment, so each patient must be evaluated and treated individually. There is no *one* solution that will work for everyone.

10. Hand-crafting The Corona Cocktails by combining low to average doses of various medications to address the multifaceted nature of neurochemical imbalances works best for most patients. I refer to this as the *rational polypharmacy* approach.

11. Primary care doctors are best suited to treat patients that need help with mood disorders and neurochemical imbalances. Many people avoid psychologists and psychiatrists for a variety of reasons, including the outdated stigma attached to seeing a "shrink," cost, availability, and trust or comfort level. Primary care doctors understand mood and the body, so they are in an ideal position to implement a complete *mind-body* treatment plan. Furthermore, given the overwhelming number of patients who need this kind of help, there are simply not enough psychiatrists to treat them all. However, I do not discourage patients from seeing professional counselors and there are many cases in which talk therapy is also necessary to make the full turn to a well-ordered life.

12. Physicians that understand how to implement this approach can help you make the most of the medications that are now on the market. In fact, it is possible that you will read about a medication in this book and realize it is exactly the supplement your body needs.

13. There is significant value for patients to understand why medications are sometimes necessary to restore emotional and physical health, what the various medications do in the brain, and what neurotransmitters are affected by those medications. Patients will also find it helpful to know why medications are effective in relieving a number of common disorders, including depression, anxiety, Attention Deficit Disorder (ADD), bipolar disorder and eating disorders.

14. The multiple symptoms related to neurochemical imbalances will open your eyes to many physical and emotional ailments that you never knew had their origins in the brain. You will learn to identify symptoms and clusters of symptoms that are likely caused by particular neurochemical imbalances.

15. You will learn my story and how I became an expert in the field of psychotropic medications and mood disorders. I will also explain why most other doctors are unaware of what the most recent and best medications are capable of doing for their patients.

16. The last chapter is a bridge to my next book in this series, which is still primarily meant for patients but I hope that doctors are also interested in both of them. The third book in this series is meant primarily for doctors, but I'm

> hoping that it will also be helpful to patients as a reliable resource guide that they and their physicians can follow. The release of this book and this series will thankfully allow me the opportunity to teach doctors how to properly use The Corona Protocol in their practices, which is easy to learn and is a lot of fun at the same time. In the last chapter I will explain what I mean by the art and science of medicine and why this field is neither one nor the other, but a fascinating symbiotic combination of both.

Having this foundation under our feet, we are now ready to frame our understanding of the mind-body connection and how we can work with it to correct the problems that are causing so much unnecessary suffering in our lives and throughout our society. There is no longer any reason that those who are sick and tired of being sick and tired are not able to get the help they need and thus have hope once again when the Protocol is fine-tuned and perfected.

CHAPTER TWO

MYTHS AND MISCONCEPTIONS

The one primary reason why more people do not know the remarkable benefits of mood-normalizing medications and why the practice of rational polypharmacology is not widespread is due to the numerous myths and misconceptions that circulate in society and are often sensationalized by the misinformed media and government. A veritable mountain of misinformation stands firmly in the way of invaluable progress. In fact, the science of this field of medicine is far more advanced than the prevailing opinion, which is, for the most part, still in the darkness of the past—in the shadow of the foreboding mountain of myths.

Having evaluated tens of thousands of patients during my practice, I am painfully aware of the myths and misconceptions that keep people from making inquiries regarding mood-normalizing medications. So before we can make significant progress in addressing chemical imbalances and their consequences, we have to get past the mountain. When it comes to our well-being, it is best not to climb the mountain or skirt around it, but to blow the damn thing to hell. We can see that the mountain has been around for a long time, weathered many storms, and has been strengthened by some of our most honored social institutions.

What are the most common and disastrous myths that are preventing people from seeking optimum health?

Myth #1: Taking Medications Indicates Weakness of Character

The misconception implicit in this myth is that a neurochemical imbalance is something that a person can control through sheer willpower. I am sure you have heard the pep talks of wannabe coaches, "Stop griping; others have it much worse than you," "What are you whining for? Just look at the sky!" "Why can't you just pull yourself together?" "Just pick yourself up by your bootstraps and move on," "What doesn't kill you makes you stronger," "I know exactly how you feel, I got real discouraged one time," and the one I hate most, "Where's your smile?" usually said with a syrupy sweet voice.

Obviously these comments do not even come close to a clinical assessment of the patient's condition or take into account the possibility of neurochemical imbalances as a cause that lies outside of our control. These are merely platitudes that have the effect of intensifying the patient's despair of getting better, because they add stress and guilt to their condition.

A related myth is implied when someone—and in this case it may even be a family doctor—says, "You realize, don't you, that this is all in your head?" or "There is no real cause for your complaints, so this is apparently a mental problem." Now to say that the problem is in the patient's head is only half right. What do you mean by mental? Aren't you referring to the brain? I'd say that's a pretty vital organ of the body, don't you think?

The physical symptoms in other parts of the body—the pain, fatigue, respiratory problems, and so on—are all real and located exactly where the patient feels them, but the original source of those symptoms lies in the fact that the neurochemicals in the brain are not doing their job. No human is able to *positive think, will power,* or *cognitive therapy* their way out of a chemical imbalance.

Previous generations knew nothing of neurochemicals and assumed they had no choice but to suffer. There was, in a sense, a certain nobility regarding suffering. The discovery of neurochemicals, however, has changed things forever and resulted in the production of the modern medications available today. Now that we know better, we need to take advantage of these amazing advances in modern science.

Myth #2: TAKING MEDICATION IS A "CRUTCH"

This next myth is closely related to the first one. Some people will tell you that only the weak person needs to take something to feel better. The truth, however, is that a chemical imbalance is a real physical cause of many disorders, and medications would not work if that were not so. They only fix a problem if there is a problem to fix. If it doesn't work, then I have chosen the wrong class of medication or I may need to reconsider the diagnosis and treatment plan. I keep practicing until I get it right. There are few people who would argue that only a weak-willed person would undergo surgery, take antibiotics or insulin and thyroid medications, and that these medications are "crutches."

Men tend to have a greater resistance to getting the help they need, partly because they have the greatest difficulty thinking something might be wrong with them. We like to believe that we can handle anything life can dish out, and from the time we were boys we have been taught to carry responsibility, be independent, and if we experience pain or suffering, to tough it out. I have found that fewer women are as intimidated as men when it comes to recognizing and dealing with a problem, but that does not mean they do not struggle with the idea that they need help. Therefore, they may be just as likely to resist going right away to see a doctor, even when they have suffered depression for a long time.

Some of my patients have felt guilty for feeling so much better after receiving proper treatment. They think that there is something wrong with taking pills to feel better, as if they were hooked on illegal drugs. Mood-normalizing medications do not work like mind-altering drugs, but merely assist the brain to function normally. Soon, after patients get used to the ease of treatment and their improved outlook on life, their guilt, hopefully, disappears. I do my best to help them understand that the benefits they are experiencing result from safe and effective medications being properly administered to actually address the underlying problem.

There are plenty of "crutches" and "Band-Aid" types of medications available that only treat symptoms, such as tranquilizers, sleeping pills and pain pills. Psychotropic medications, however, are different. They actually fix the underlying problems that the body can't fix itself. These medications do not merely cover up problems. They cure them. This is why I refer to them as preventative and the most holistic substances available. Their one purpose is to help the body heal itself, which is what holistic health is all about.

Myth #3: MOOD-NORMALIZING MEDICATIONS ARE ADDICTIVE

Everyone knows that it is possible to get "hooked" on pain medications or some other prescription drug—such as amphetamines, tranquilizers (benzodiazepines) and barbiturates, which are legally used as sedatives, to control pain, and so on. This class of medications is referred to as *controlled substances* that are regulated by the government, require a special triplicate prescription, and they can be abused. It needs to be absolutely clear that the medications described in this book and that have proven to be most useful in treating mood are entirely nonaddictive. The only possible exception applies to patients whose symptoms indicate that they have ADD or ADHD (Attention Deficit Hyperactive Disorder). In these cases a stimulant may be prescribed in appropriate doses, and patients can be closely monitored. If stimulants are taken for the wrong reasons, they can be addictive. If they are taken appropriately for treatment of ADD/ADHD, then the risk of addiction is minimal.

The fact is, many of these patients at one time or another had been *self-medicating* without knowing it through the illegal use of drugs, and were, therefore, doing more harm than good to themselves. One of the remarkable benefits of antidepressant, antianxiety, and ADD-related medications is that they relieve the brain's perceived need for narcotics. In fact, some patients report that after beginning a regimen of mood-normalizing medications, they spontaneously gave up cigarettes, alcohol and illicit drugs because they no longer felt the need for them.

People do not usually have concerns over the addictive potential of other prescribed medications, such as in treating a rash, infection, or other "real" medical problems. When it comes to a chemical imbalance, most doctors and patients prefer to merely treat symptoms rather than take a proactive approach to *preventing the symptoms*. Mood-normalizing medications restore normalcy to the brain and nervous system and are effective only in cases where they are needed. If it were possible to be addicted to feeling normal, then I suppose that would be the one addiction I would not worry about.

Myth #4: Mood-Normalizing Medications Require Weeks or Months to Work

The conventional approach to treating a mood disorder with medications is to begin with one particular medication and gradually increase the dosage. This approach has proven to be an ineffective and haphazard way to practice this field of medicine, which requires creativity and a lot of practice. The results of this method of titrating one medication, such as an SSRI, slowly from low to high dose are incomplete, intensify the negative side-effects, and require a "wait and see" period of time to determine how the patient responds. The correct approach is to first make the best assessment possible, based on what can be learned about the patient's neurophysiology, symptoms, and background, then determine what neurochemicals would be responsible for causing the symptoms and treat them with the appropriate medication or combination of medications to restore the patient's chemical balance in the most efficient and effective way with the fewest side effects.

Amazingly, lower to average doses of mood normalizing medications, and using them in combination to address all the specific chemical issues, consistently produce better and faster results. This is, in fact, the essence of my rational polypharmaceutical method. The misconception is that medications *necessarily* require weeks before the patient begins to show signs of improvement, but the reality is that if it is the right medication it works quickly, usually within days to at most two weeks. If there is no improvement in that period of time, the patient should not be given higher doses of a medication that already does not work, but should be started on something else. The reason for making the switch, as we will see in a later chapter, is that there is more than one chemical involved in positive, normal feelings. If the results are just okay, or side effects outweigh the benefits, then there is most likely a better choice available.

Myth #5: Unpleasant Side Effects Are Acceptable

Side effects, unless short-term and mild, should not be tolerated by either the doctor or the patient. If patients complain about negative side effects of the medication they are taking, I listen closely to what they have to say and then, based on specific complaints, I can almost always find an alternative that produces the results we desire without significant side effects. The only exception to this rule that I would tolerate is if there were no suitable alternative and the patient was willing to put up with minor side effects for the greater benefit of normal health.

There are some side effects that are erased merely by the combination of medications required to treat the problem. However, I do not advocate adding a medication for the sake of treating side effects of the original medication. For example, giving a sleeping pill to deal with insomnia caused by a medication, or giving a stimulant to combat fatigue is not usually, in my opinion, the best approach. Significant side effects generally serve as a signal that the wrong neurochemical is being targeted, the dosage is too high, or it is simply not the right medication for that person.

The situation in which one medication could be added that would resolve the side effects of another agent would be when the first medication is not the *cause* of the side effects, but has *uncovered* symptoms which previously existed but were masked by a variety of other symptoms. Combining medications takes advantage of the strengths of each and avoids the weaknesses that result from using any one medication that is tapered up too high. *Rational Poly-pharmacology* produces the best of both worlds.

Myth #6: Mood-Normalizing Medications Should Only Be Used Briefly

The flip side of this misconception is that once people begin taking a medication, they will have to take it for the rest of their lives. Neither statement is true. Because of the variables of each person's nervous system, it is impossible at the outset to determine how long the patient will need to use the medications. The answer to this question is not up to either the patient or doctor, but is up to the patient's body. We need to listen to what our bodies are telling us. We may have our opinions about what is right or wrong, but frankly your body doesn't care about your opinions. It just wants to feel better.

There are several factors that can help guide us in determining how long is long enough:

a. If genetics plays a greater role in the patient's imbalance, then the most benefit will come through a longer stretch of time. The stronger the link to one's parents or other family members, the longer it will take for the body to learn how to balance its neurochemicals on its own.

b. If the patient has suffered from a mood disorder for a long time, a longer medical treatment will usually be required.

c. The more traumatic (psychologically, physically, sexually) the physical cause of a chemical imbalance is will also be a determining factor as to how long one will be on medications. If the patient does not receive counseling from a qualified psychologist, then even more time can be added to their required use of medication.

d. If the circumstances of the patient's life are especially stress-inducing, then the ongoing use of medication will also likely be helpful.

e. The body goes through chemical changes during certain seasons of our lives and those changes can be from moderate to radical—for men, normal seasons of change include puberty and "middle age" (their forties and fifties), and for women they are puberty, postpartum (after having children), and mid to late thirties, forties and fifties. Tapering off of medications during times of hormonal changes may result in the recurrence of previous symptoms for some.

In general, after "full remission" (when chemical balance has been restored and patients feel like their old selves again or are feeling better than any other time in their lives), the patient may continue on medication for six months to a year or so and then slowly taper off, provided that there is nothing in their environment creating an unusual amount of stress. Again, these are artificial time frames, and the body does not care how long it is as long as it is long enough. The extended and tapering off periods give patients the opportunity to assess their health and well being, and provide their brains adequate time to fully adjust to the new and healthy state. Before I begin to decrease their medication, I review my patients' history and remind them how they felt prior to using the medication, since they may have forgotten all the details after feeling better for a while. This discussion is meant to alert them to symptoms they need to watch for as the medications are tapered down and eventually stopped.

Some patients will settle into a low dose of medication for life, because they find a *threshold* dose, and when they drop below it, symptoms may begin to reoccur. These doses may not have been adequate at the beginning of their treatment, which proves the curative properties of the medications they have received and that in responding to those medications, the body has repaired itself.

Patients need to understand that if we begin to reduce the dosage of their medications, but find we have to return to a full dose to maintain the best results, it is not their fault and they have not done anything wrong, but their bodies are not ready to function normally on their own yet. By way of analogy, some people suffer from allergies and other people do not. The factor that determines whether they react to pollen or cat dander, for example, is the uniqueness of their particular immune system.

Myth #7: MOOD-NORMALIZING MEDICATIONS ARE DANGEROUS

I will not downplay potential risks of mood-normalizing medications, but the fact is that there is no danger to the average person when these medications are properly prescribed and administered. Side effects are generally mild and self-limited, and eventually disappear. If any side effect is significant, the medication may be stopped. Of the multiple thousands of patients I've seen during more than two decades of practice, I have not encountered any serious, significant, or persistent side effects. Neither have I seen a single death resulting from their use. There is no evidence of any long-term damage caused by these medications and usually no blood monitoring if needed, other than basic regular screening labs for diabetes, kidney and liver function, electrolytes, blood count, thyroid function, cholesterol, etc. These medications do not cause damage to the organs or any other permanent damage to any area of the body. The potential benefits way outweigh the potential risks.

In this area of medicine, in a sense, we need to work backwards. We make educated guesses as to which imbalances need to be corrected. We discover whether we were right only after the fact, by determining whether the desired results were achieved. When I choose the wrong medication, or combination of medications, the feedback I receive from the patient points me in the right direction. Side effects are, therefore, a necessary factor in the diagnosis and treatment of the disorder. Thankfully, the positive effects of the proper combination and dosage are greater than any side effects, and that is the ultimate goal we are trying to achieve.

Myth #8: Alcohol Must Not be Consumed While On Medication

Too much alcohol is dangerous and physically destructive, especially to the nervous system, under any circumstances. Drinking to excess destroys brain cells and can interfere with prescription drugs or intensify their negative side effects. Alcoholics and pregnant women should not drink any alcohol ever under any circumstances. Excessive drinking also disrupts the normal mind-body balance, increasing the symptoms of mood disorders.

Most "social drinkers" can tolerate a moderate intake of alcohol while on medications, but they should heed the warning on the label to avoid driving and should not operate heavy equipment. Otherwise it would be unrealistic to assume that the average patient would discontinue drinking entirely, and if they were told to give up alcohol, some would be less willing to accept treatment.

A few patients have told me that they do not take their medications when they are planning on going out and drinking. However, I would rather they take their meds anyway, because that may help them have the presence of mind to not overdo it. A person who enjoys a proper balance of neurochemicals is less likely to abuse alcohol. In fact, there is nothing more wonderful and delightfully intoxicating than life itself when the brain is in good working order.

My observations about the interaction of mood-normalizing medications and alcohol are:

a. For some people, medications increase sensitivity to alcohol. One drink may affect them the way two drinks did without medication, and two drinks may affect them like three to four. I joke with some of my patients that this makes for cheaper dates. I want my patients to know when to say, "No thank you, I've had enough."

b. Excessive drinking can decrease the effectiveness of the medications. In fact, the patient may find that their mood worsens after they have been drinking, and this is also true of marijuana use, because THC (tetrahydrocannabinol, the psychoactive ingredient in marijuana) is a known depressant and can last in the body and continue to affect the nervous system for up to a month. People who live with a family member who abuses alcohol or uses marijuana can tell you about the "day after," when the user is grouchier than usual and unhappy about almost everything.

Myth #9: Medications Should not be Taken During Pregnancy or Breast-feeding

There is an element of truth in this statement, but it is not absolutely true. Each woman needs to be individually assessed to determine her needs and those of her unborn child. In most cases, the potential risks are minimal and the potential gains are great, so the doctor should strongly consider medications during pregnancy if they are needed. A deciding factor will be the mother's mental and emotional state if she is off her medications and the potential harm to the child if she does not take medications that may be good for her.

Nevertheless, there is no harm in cutting back the normal dosage for a pregnant woman to see how she responds. I usually try to taper down and off medications at some point during pregnancy to see if they are still needed, maybe about the end of the first trimester and beginning of the second trimester, more or less, and this individualized treatment approach has been successful for the vast majority of my patients. Again, this is up to the woman's body. Some women are affected by the radical hormonal changes of pregnancy for the better and other women for the worse. Since the estrogen level is very high during pregnancy, and hormones are not fluctuating as they normally would, this can create a more stable balance for some women. I have heard some women say, "I've never felt better than when I was pregnant," and some women experience the "pregnancy glow."

In my many years of treating women during pregnancy and breast-feeding, I have never seen any significant negative effect to either mother or child produced by mood-normalizing medications. Psychotropic medications typically release inactive metabolites into the breast milk, which means that there is no active medication that passes through the breast milk. This can be researched, and it is important to openly discuss this with your doctor and other hopefully reliable sources of information. Treatment decisions can then be individualized.

It is possible that the child may fare better if the mother is emotionally healthy during the pregnancy and breast-feeding. In the end, healthier mothers and healthier babies should be among the major goals when treating the population anyway.

Myth #10: MEDICATIONS SHOULD NOT BE PRESCRIBED FOR CHILDREN AND ADOLESCENTS

Adolescents go through a major transition during puberty in which their bodies are chemically altered with the onset of adulthood. Parents have seen huge personality changes occur almost overnight, as their teenager becomes more irritable, less interested in the family, and sleeping more than usual. Add to the chemical changes, the hardships many young people endure in the socialization that goes on when attending junior high and high school, and it becomes clear why the first signs of depression often appear during adolescence and why suicide is the number three cause of death among teenagers.

Based on my experience with mood-normalizing medications and their beneficial use with young people, I would oppose any sort of age discrimination in their administration. In my practice, these medications have been proven to be safe and well tolerated by young people when prescribed correctly. The results can be excellent, and often come easier and are better than in those who are over the age of eighteen. Since their brains do not have the long period of conditioning of older patients, they are more responsive to treatment.

Mood-normalizing medications should be prescribed for children and adolescents in the same fashion as for everyone else, and, if anything, should parallel treatment of the elderly, which means the "low and slow approach." Again, each person's nervous system is unique, so I find some adults do well with pediatric doses and some children do better with "adult" doses. The medication response does not depend as much on age, size and sex as one would think. The numbers aren't important, rather it's the results that count and matter. The response seems to be more genetically determined and has to do with how well an individual metabolizes certain products.

I especially enjoy working with children and adolescents, because making a positive difference in their lives prepares them for a brighter future. They can be spared years of suffering that their parents and ancestors had to endure. With the right treatment, we also increase the chances that they will make better choices regarding their behavior and decisions.

Parents who feel guilty about giving their children mood-normalizing medications need to get over it. In most cases, the parent is merely embarrassed that "something is wrong with their child," when in fact chemical imbalances are so prevalent that they are the norm rather than the exception. A loving parent will take whatever steps are necessary to ensure the health, safety and well-being of the child.

Myth #11: Mood-Normalizing Medications Increase Risk of Suicide

A few years ago the government issued a "black box warning" about an increased risk of suicide for children and adolescents, and more recently young adults, taking antidepressant medications. The warning, however, was based on faulty logic and inadequate research. In actual fact, the suicide rate had dramatically decreased since the first modern antidepressant, Prozac (Fluoxetine), was introduced. In time, the government warning actually led to more suicides because the fear it created caused some people to discontinue taking their antidepressants. I predicted that would happen when this warning was issued, and, unfortunately, I was right. Also, doctors are more hesitant. Parents of children and adolescents are hesitant. Patients themselves are hesitant, and this has created an unnecessary environment of fear and suspicion. The unfortunate reality is that this false warning by our federal government has led to the first substantial and sustained suicide rate increase in over 20 years, since Prozac was introduced.

The confusion by the government is that the studies they relied on to reach this decision revealed no actual completed suicides. The studies noted very rare "suicidal thinking," and the government made the confusing leap that these medications caused increased suicidal thinking for most people, but that's simply not true. In actuality the exact opposite is true. Suicidal thinking was symptomatic of the depression that originally resulted in patients taking antidepressants.

The government tends to not look at people as individuals, but as a group. The individuals that make up that group, however, may not be very closely related. The government paints things with one broad stroke, though I've found that the individual needs a much softer and more detailed stroke. The basic confusion surrounding this issue is that if antidepressants are given to someone with bipolar disorder, there is a risk of inducing mania, with the potential risk of increased suicidal thinking and behavior. This is a valid concern, but the physician who knows what he or she is doing will assess and monitor the patient, and if bipolar disorder is evident, respond with the appropriate medication. Even the mood stabilizers that treat bipolar disorder have a suicide warning on them, which is ridiculous.

One big problem is that government, and most doctors in general, do not know how to distinguish depression and anxiety disorders ("unipolar" disorders) from bipolar disorder. The average psychiatrist requires seven to ten years with a client to properly diagnose bipolar disorder. If this is the case with the "specialists", it explains why it is a source of confusion with most doctors, the government, and society in general. Unipolar disorders are much more common than bipolar disorders, but a bipolar disorder is still fairly common (about ten percent or more of the population) and has been tragically under-diagnosed. Therefore, the general population needs better information about these various disorders and how they should be treated.

Moving Mountains

I hope that by now you are at least enlightened and interested in the awesome results people experience with mood-normalizing meds (if not totally enchanted). At least we have turned the mountain of myths and misconceptions to a pile of rubble, so now we can continue down the pathway of discovery. If you are ready to take that next step, unencumbered by the falsehoods that you once carried, and enter a better life and discover a new and improved you in a world of beauty and joy, then it is my pleasure to serve as your guide.

HEALING
— THE —
MIND AND BODY
VOLUME 1
SECOND EDITION

— SECTION II —

- THE TECHNOLOGY OF MOODS
- NEUROTRANSMITTERS: THE BRAIN'S CHEMISTRY SET
- "I'M NOT A PILL PERSON"

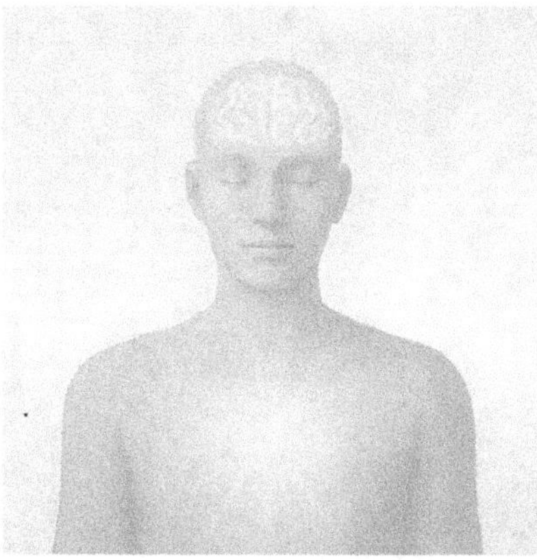

PAUL D. CORONA, M.D.

CHAPTER THREE

THE TECHNOLOGY OF MOODS

PHYSICAL CAUSE – MENTAL SYMPTOMS

What do you think, Dr. Paul, Am I depressed?" Ben put this question to me during a physical exam required by his insurance company. In response, I asked him to list and describe his symptoms. I asked if he was aware of any *physical* changes or other symptoms in his body and told him we would analyze his bloodwork and other test results. Then we talked about depression and how it can grow in the mind as a result of life experiences—such as early conditioning, a persistent feeling of helplessness and powerlessness, and so on—or as a result of natural chemical changes to which we are all subject as we age. We agreed on starting him on a treatment program even before we saw the lab results of his blood test, because I have learned that a medication trial is the most reliable diagnostic tool and it has the advantage of excluding the need for more extensive lab work and testing.

What does it mean when someone says, "I'm feeling depressed?" What happens within the human brain that creates moods, such as depression, anxiety, rage, or even our positive feelings? What *physical situation* translates into mental states and vice versa, and how is that situation resolved by administering medication? In asking this question, notice that we are approaching the issue of mood disorders with a different strategy than a psychologist would adopt. The psychotherapist would probe life events for trauma or childhood programming and how that shaped the patients internal belief system, or notion of reality—especially their self-perception based on their absolute beliefs, even if the patient is not conscious of those beliefs and how they affect outlook, mood, behavior, and so on. The role of the counselor is to assist the person in uncovering those hidden beliefs. The counselor should also rationally analyze them, discover where and why they are and explain how the wrong beliefs negatively affect the patient, and then work at *reprogramming* their thinking to develop a healthier outlook on life. Eventually the feelings of depression may diminish until they are completely eradicated in some patients.

As a physician, I ask a different set of questions that are designed to locate the physical and neurochemical causes of depression. My education and training concentrates on the mental health of a person as a thinking *organism*, how the organism functions and malfunctions, and how to treat it when a malfunction occurs. My job, therefore, is to balance and normalize these delicate neurological systems.

I hope it is clear that I do not think of my patients as nothing more than a collection of functioning parts within an organic body, because I am, in fact, saying exactly the opposite. My concern for the *person* is what compels me to use what I know in my own area of specialization to look for physical causes of emotional complaints. Psychologists and physicians are concerned with the same problems, but we take different points of view and adopt different strategies. As I have said, there are many cases in which the best results occur as a result of patient, doctor, and psychologist working together on the patient's behalf. It is also true that many people are not going to improve, no matter how much psychotherapy they receive, if the physical condition does not receive due consideration and treatment.

If you understand computers, then think of the brain as the *hardware* of our mind where all of our thinking and feeling processes occur. The *software* would then be the specific patterns, associations, and methods we develop for analyzing all the incoming data. We also need certain resident programs built into the hardware so that the neural computer can carry out functions without creating huge demands on our conscious functions—such as breathing, adjusting body temperature, heart rate, etc.

Given this model of the brain, which certainly has its weaknesses when we begin actual comparisons with computers, doctors and neurologists are trained to troubleshoot any problems with the *hardware* while psychologists are trained to analyze and tweak the *software*, or *programming*. A problem with the *hardware* (the brain) means the *software* programs will not run properly. Depression and other mood disorders are like the error message of our neural computer that warns us when something goes wrong.

A serious roadblock to psychotherapy is that by the time a patient finally enlists the help of a counselor, the brain has had enough time to reinforce neural pathways that reinforce the negative or problematic thinking and suppress the distribution of chemicals that would otherwise enable the person to ward off depression or otherwise function normally. Of course, the irony is that the very condition that requires attention and healing sabotages the process by disabling the patient at the source. In these cases, medications are the most effective means of bringing the patient to a point where he can think and act clearly and freely enough to go to work on the other psychological issues. In fact, with regard to specific mood disorders, medications are not only the best remedy, but also the only remedy that works, or at least works the best.

When I take the time to explain to patients how their brains work and the "mechanics" of neurology, how it can go wrong, and why that results in depression, anxiety, bipolar disorders, eating disorders, and other similar problems, they are often relieved and say something like, "OK, then you're saying I'm not crazy?" They are actually pleased to learn that the problem is in the physical functions of their bodies and can be "fixed."

So now I am going to do for you what I do for all of my patients: Take you on a quick tour through some of the components of a normal brain so that you will have a basic understanding of how it works. There is no need to be worried, because you will not need a medical degree to follow what I am about to teach and show you.

The Brain: The Infinitesimal Universe

Think for a moment of all the functions your brain constantly performs (by the way, your brain never sleeps, but it puts you to sleep so it can perform needed repairs and adjustments without you distracting it or getting in its way). Every part of your body, every organ, and all of your tissues, need constant monitoring and regulation. For example, looking at just one vital system in this whole complex structure, the adrenals begin to produce cortisol about an hour before you wake up each morning. This chemical boost helps you to get out of bed and started into your day. By the afternoon, however, that cortisol production shuts down. Otherwise you would not be able to fall asleep each night, and that is what accounts for the drop in energy we often experience mid-afternoon (great time for a nap).

Cortisol is merely one of many chemicals your body has to produce, adjust, and balance to maintain physical equilibrium, which we call "homeostasis." In fact the whole array of factors that must be constantly managed by the brain is overwhelming; the immune system, thyroid gland, liver, kidneys, and so on. Nevertheless, the central headquarters for handling all of these processes is contained in a relatively small area in the human brain.

At the same time, without your "knowledge," your brain is enabling your body to survive, protect, and nourish itself, and get around your need to be aware of what is going on in your external environment. All the challenges that you must assess and address, including air temperature, potential danger, anticipations of what might happen next, and even carrying out simple movements like scratching an itch, are all accomplished at the same time. While dealing with all of this, your brain is working at perception, analysis, storage and retrieval of all the information that is bombarding your senses. The brain of self-conscious beings, such as ourselves, also observes various feelings and makes decisions regarding what to do about those feelings. (Yes, that *is* a lot of work!)

Nerve Cell or Neuron

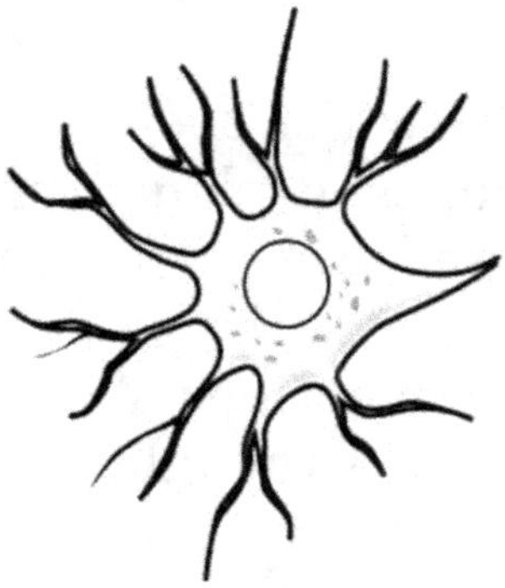

Our tour through the brain will focus mostly on its smallest components and their functions: The nerve cells or *neurons*.

Simply to get started, think of *neurons* as tiny light bulbs on a map. No neuron fires on its own, but they light up in clusters located in the same region of the brain, with a few communication lines to other clusters in other regions of the brain.

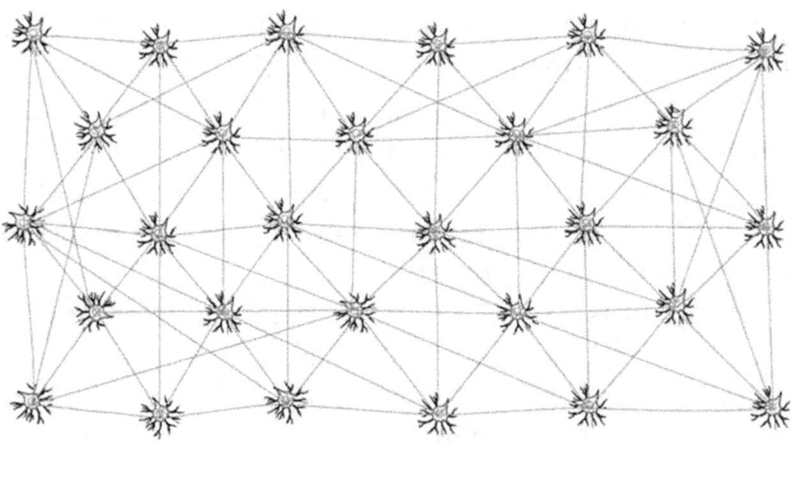

Think of the brain as an electrical system with a complicated mesh of wires that seem to flow endlessly. The nervous system is composed of over 100 billion neurons which are visible only through powerful microscopes. Each neuron connects with at least one thousand other cells, which means that the communication grid has a potential of more than too trillion connections. And yet it takes less than one second for a thought to register in the brain while engaging millions of neurons. The chemicals travel around the nervous system about 1,000 times every second throughout one's life. It's difficult for the human brain to comprehend these numbers.

Neurons are all pretty much the same. Neurons do not store information, such as how to spell the word *stop* correctly or what you ate for breakfast yesterday. Rather, the essence of a memory exists within a pattern of the *interaction of specific neurons* when triggered in a cluster. Each cluster is the segment of an event, such as thoughts, feelings, decision-making, and movements. As you read this sentence, millions of clusters (like tiny neighborhoods) are lighting up all over your brain with relays that connect them together. Some clusters are dedicated to size and shape, others to color, others to texture, and so on.

The clusters of neurons that correspond to your experience of an object are spread throughout the brain. For example, think of a rose. Your visual experience occurs in a separate area of your

NEURON

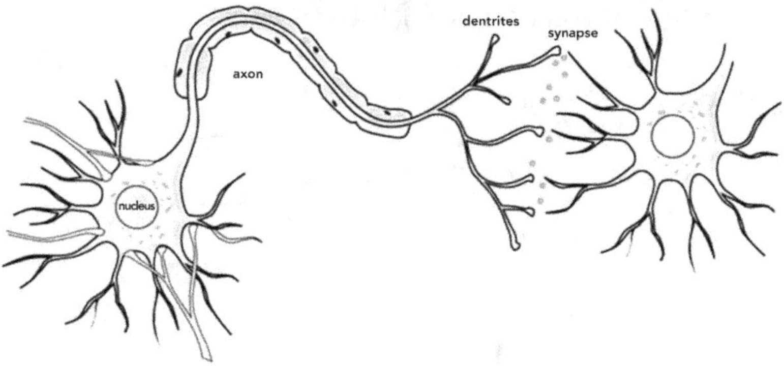

brain from that of smell, which is separated from the area that accounts for sensations of touch. If you pick up the rose—or even *think* of picking it up—a different area of your brain is activated. Nevertheless, these various locations of neural activity act together in perfect harmony.

A *neuron* sends a signal through a wire-like filament called the *axon*. They *receive* messages through tiny branches (*dendrites*) that spread out in all directions. Imagine a complicated mesh of telephone lines that enable neurons to "talk to each other." A neuron sends an impulse through its axon, which is received by another neuron through one of its dendrites.

These incredibly thin wires, however, do not actually touch each other, but are separated by a tiny gap known as a *synapse*. If one wire is sending information to another, something has to happen at the synapse level in order to carry

Enlarged view of synapse-gap

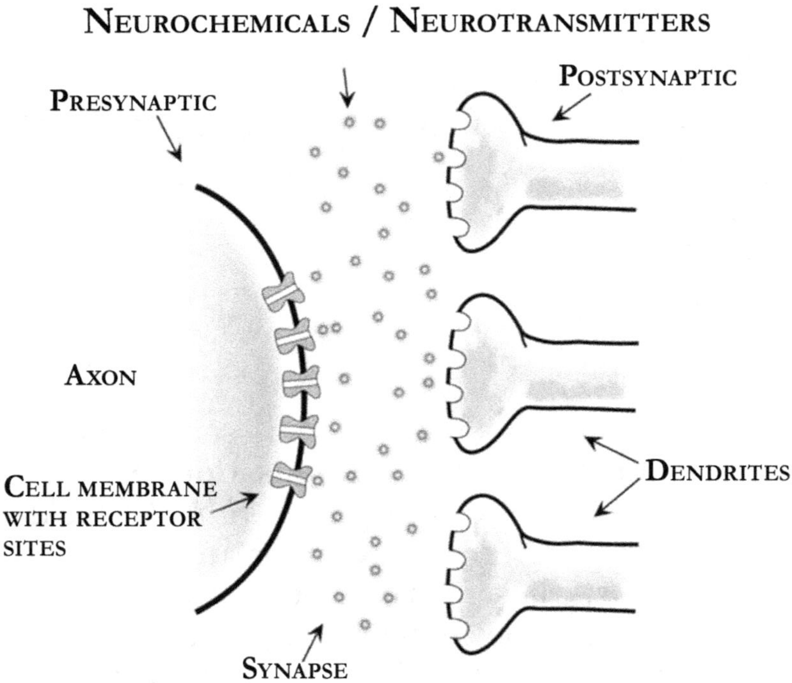

that information forward. What happens is the release of a neurochemical by one wire into the gap where it is then taken up by the other wire. In the

Ideal Neurons

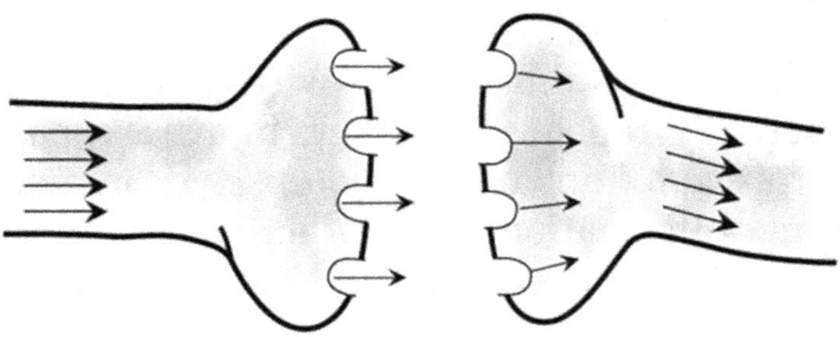

following diagram, the small circles represent the neurochemicals inside the synapse (gap) between the nerve cells. This illustration shows the ideal communication between two nerve cells that are functioning properly.

The side of the gap that *transmits (sends)* the

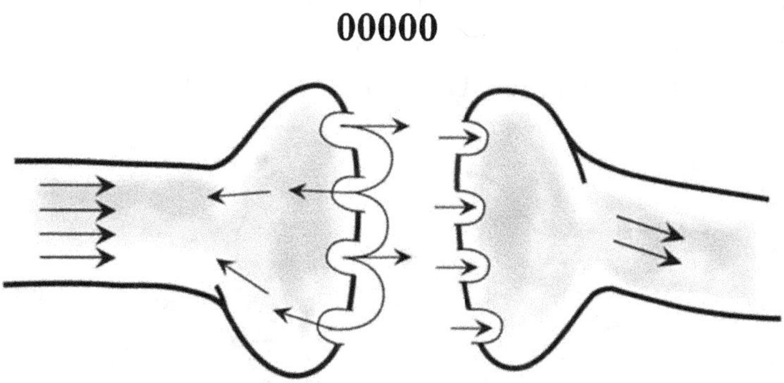

neurochemicals is referred to as *presynaptic*. These chemicals are passed through the cell membrane by way of small holes called *receptors*. The side that *receives,* or *uptakes,* the neurochemicals on the transmitter cell is referred to as *postsynaptic*. The chemicals pass through other receptors in the cell membrane of the next neuron. Each receptor site has a specific function, and only certain neurochemicals are allowed to pass through certain receptor sites.

Unfortunately, the nerve cells do not always communicate successfully across the synapse. The receptor sites the chemicals travel through should ideally transmit the chemicals in one direction—forward.

Imbalances in the nervous system occur when the receptor sites *spring a leak,* allowing the chemicals to move in the wrong direction—backward. The neurochemicals therefore fail to pass through the nerves efficiently, causing an imbalance that affects whatever tissue is at the end of that nerve. This leakage is detrimental to the purpose and function of neurochemicals, because they are not allowed to continue the forward flow of commu-

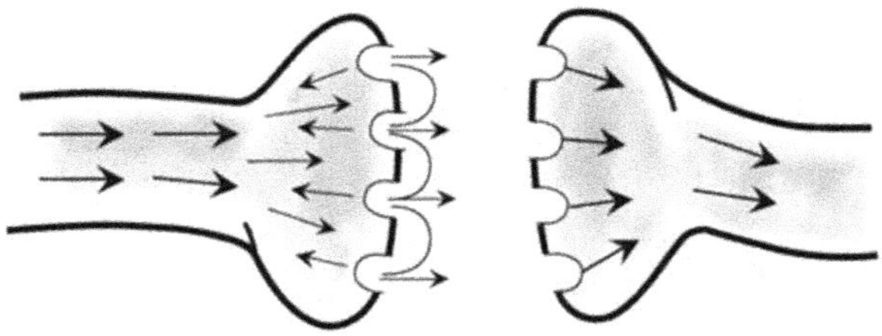

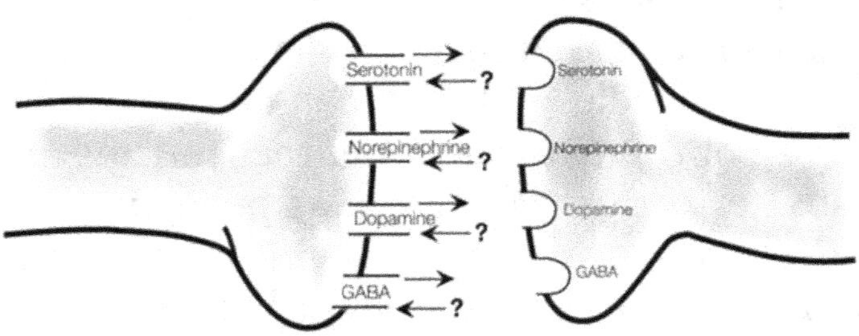

Multiple Neurochemical Imbalances

nication from one neuron to the next. When the neurotransmitter is one of the chemicals related to feelings of well-being and happiness, the results can produce a large number of unwanted consequences in both the mind (emotions, feelings, etc.) and body. Even if some chemicals travel normally, but others do not, the health of the entire body can be adversely affected. When many chemicals are not moving along as they should, the mental and physical breakdowns will be more numerous and more severe.

The flow of chemicals in the synapse begins at the axon and travels to the dendrites where they are absorbed to continue the relay from one neuron to another. At any given time, a number of different chemicals—serving a variety of functions—will be present in the synapse, but always making that same forward progress and moving only in one direction if they are functioning in an ideal fashion.

In order to pass through the receptor site and into the end of the dendrite, cell membranes are equipped with ions, such as calcium and sodium. Now as long as every chemical is traveling through the nerve cells correctly, the brain and body are harmonized and yield optimal health. If there is any defect in the system, however, the neurochemicals will not move normally through the synapses, which causes the chemicals to imbalance, preventing the brain from operating effectively. Neurochemicals that are forced to sit around in the *synaptic soup* wait for a gate to open up somewhere so they can move on. Perhaps they finally move in the right direction into the next nerve cell, or maybe they are drawn back into the axon that released them, which in turn causes a malfunction in the nervous system since this is the wrong way for them to move. The breakdown in the communication across the synapse will affect other parts of the body that are not receiving the attention they deserve or that are forced to carry additional stress.

To appreciate the importance of the delicate balance of chemicals in the brain, we need to remind ourselves of the direct and dynamic connection of the brain to the body. In other words, the problems resulting from an imbalance are not only periodic or chronic mood disorders. Organs, glands and tissues of the body are also subject to excessive stress. Organs and glands have their own chemical properties and functions, which may introduce further imbalances. For example, the adrenal glands may release a surge of cortisol, which can cause a surge of epinephrine (adrenaline). An excess of cortisol—usually due to mental stress and anxiety—has been linked to bone disease, such as osteoporosis. An excess of epinephrine can weaken the immune system and leave the body more susceptible to disease.

In the next chapter I will introduce you to the primary neurochemicals (the small circles in the previous illustration) that we know are associated with positive feelings such as joy, pleasure, and simply being in a good mood. To prepare you, here are their names: *serotonin, norepinephrine, dopamine* and *GABA* (gamma-aminobutyric acid). There are may other chemicals and factors, such as glutamate, glycine, histamine, acetylcholine, electrolytes like sodium and calcium, and others. However, I will focus my discussion on "The Big 4" for the sake of simplicity. Remember, these are simply the labels we have given to specific chemicals that are present in the brain and throughout the rest of the nervous system, and they are nothing more than that. Even though these words may be long and unfamiliar to you, there is no reason to think that you will not be able to understand what comes next. If you want to know whether you have a chemical imbalance and what that means exactly, it is going to be spelled out for you in a very simple way.

What Went Wrong?

What is a chemical imbalance? What exactly are we talking about when we say that certain neurotransmitters are not doing what they are supposed to be doing?

The short answer: Chemicals that are supposed to communicate from one neuron to another fail to make the short trip through the synaptic gap for a number of reasons. These include postsynaptic receptors that do not admit *easy access* for neurochemicals, presynaptic receptors that have been disabled or damaged by substance abuse, and sluggish movement of the chemicals. The most primary reason though is leakage of the presynaptic receptor sites (and occasionally postsynaptic receptor site problems) due to genetic predisposition, hormonal changes, outside stressors, and other factors such as environmental, etc. When all the factors come together in an individual, I refer to this as the "perfect storm." Notice that it is not the case that *insufficiency of a particular neurochemical is the cause of the imbalance.* Some people resist taking antidepressants because they do not want to "get their happiness from a pill," as if we were prescribing recreational drugs. Mood normalizing medications do not add serotonin or any of the other three neurochemicals to our nervous system, but rather bind to the nerve cells within the synapse so that *the chemicals that are already there will move and work according to their design.* The medications actually block a person's own chemicals from going back the wrong way. The necessary neurochemicals are already present, and have been present since birth. They simply need help. I think of myself as a plumber and electrician, since basically what I do all day is fix leaks and rewire neurons.

Unfortunately, many people who have mood disorders attempt to *self-medicate* with alcohol or the abuse of other substances. They do not usually know that they are self-medicating, they only know that they are not happy unless they are high, or that life is not working out well for them, or they would rather be oblivious than face all the challenges and hardships of their circumstances. Other people spend a fortune on mega-vitamins and other supplements that they have been led to believe will make them healthier and happier. Of course the list of remedies goes on and on, but unless the chemical imbalances are addressed directly, there is not a lot of hope that the brain will heal itself naturally.

Have you looked for something to do, apply, or ingest to make you feel better? If so, and you have read this far, the likelihood is that whatever else you have tried has not worked for you. So we will leave behind the supposed remedies that do not work and learn about the medications that can help you finally feel better once and for all. Let me assure you, all that your body needs for you to feel better and have a normal level of enjoyment in life is already present within your nervous system. All we have to do is find the right medication or combination of medications to restore the balance of those chemicals. Once that simple feat is accomplished, you are going to look back at your life and wonder how you ever survived living under the cloud of your former mood disorder.

Chapter Four

Neurotransmitters: The Brain's Chemistry Set

Do you trust all car mechanics? Suppose you take your car to one of those assembly line-type auto-repair shops with a coupon that entitles you to service on your car. The mechanic tinkers with your car for a while and then returns to the waiting room with the bad news. He cannot perform the service because other parts around it are either worn out or were defective from the manufacturer and are about to break, resulting in severe and expensive damage to your vehicle. However, for a small fortune, the mechanic can replace the defective parts and then perform the free service—for no additional cost. Do you trust this mechanic?

How can you protect yourself from shady mechanics, contractors, plumbers, and anyone else who might attempt to scare you into paying for unnecessary service to your property? One way is to know as much about automobiles, and yours in particular, as the mechanic knows. If you can say, "I just checked those hoses (gaskets or whatever) a couple of days ago, and there's no problem with them. Service the car like the coupon says and get me back on the road again." Another way to handle the situation is to ask as many questions as possible—a million questions if that is what it takes. "Oh, there's a problem with the hoses? Well, what do they do? What do they connect? What runs through them? How are they damaged? How can you tell?"

Why ask all these pesky questions? Because you have a right to know. If someone is going to charge you for performing a service to something that belongs to you, then you have the right to know what exactly is the problem, how that person is going to fix it, and why it is going to cost you money to have the work done. Now if this applies to your car, home, or computer, how much more would it apply to your body and your brain?

I am going to keep this chapter as short and painless as possible. Believe me, I would not even consider providing the average patient with this information if I was not completely convinced that it is of the greatest benefit for all of us to understand what can happen when one of these four chemicals is out of whack. We are going to examine each of the four neurochemicals I am focusing on, that we know are directly involved in producing either good moods or bad moods and stress-related physical symptoms, such as chronic pain disorders or any other manifestation of how the mind and body work either together or apart. I will begin each section with symptoms relating to a malfunction of the neurochemical under discussion and then list the medications that prove to be most effective in correcting those malfunctions.

But first, a warning: A big surprise may be lurking in the following pages. If you are not reading this book for your own health, but for a friend or family member, do not be shocked if in one of the lists of symptoms you recognize the very problems you have had to wrestle with from time to time. Even though it would never have occurred to you that your suffering was caused by a mood disorder, if a list or partial list matches your symptoms, you should consider having a discussion with your doctor about the medications posted here. If your doctor is unfamiliar with treating these symptoms with mood normalizing medications, then take this book with you on your next visit.

THE BIG FOUR

Since most people do not use the following words in their daily conversations, I will refresh your memory regarding the four neurochemicals that I mentioned in the previous chapter: *Serotonin, norepinephrine, dopamine, and GABA.* An important fact to note regarding these chemicals is that in the majority of patients I have treated for neurochemical imbalances, the problem cannot be traced to one of the four chemicals, but in almost every case involves a combination of two or more chemicals that are not doing their job. I refer to this condition simply as a *mixed imbalance.* Of course this comes as no surprise given the complexity of the nervous system and the way its various communication systems are interconnected and intertwined. In reality there are other chemicals and factors involved besides these four neurochemicals, but as I said before, I choose to break it down like this for simplicity so the subject is easier to understand.

In the diagram below I will attempt an illustration of what an imbalance of overlapping neurochemicals looks like:

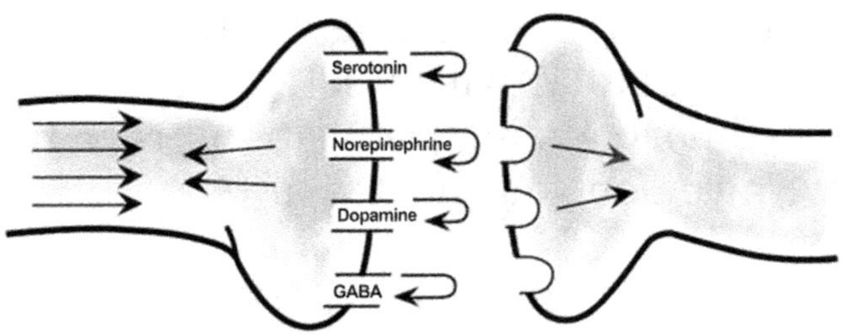

Imbalance of Overlapping Neurochemicals

1. Serotonin

If you have heard anything about neurochemicals, it is likely that serotonin is the one that has stayed in your memory. That is because serotonin has hogged the spotlight when it comes to the Big Four—which is way more attention than it deserves. In the larger scheme of chemical imbalances, serotonin often plays a minor role compared to the other neurochemicals.

Symptoms associated with serotonin imbalance include:

- Worry
- Obsessive thinking/rumination
- Depression
- Some anxiety and related symptoms
- Some physical symptoms
- Food cravings
- Sexual symptoms (i.e.: premature ejaculation, erectile dysfunction, delayed orgasm or anorgasmia (failure to achieve orgasm). In other words, no payoff at the end.
- Symptoms that have a hormonal component (i.e. PMS or other symptoms related to the luteal phase—the second half—of the menstrual cycle, postpartum, perimenopausal and menopausal).

When balancing serotonin, doctors have eight SSRIs and four SNRIs to choose from.

SSRI: Selective Serotonin Reuptake Inhibitor. These medications resolve the problem at the neuron (nerve cell) level by binding to the receptor sites (holes) and preventing the chemical serotonin from moving the wrong way, and thus this chemical is forced to move the right way, which is forward. SSRI's selectively inhibit the abnormal reuptake of serotonin, hence the name SSRI.

Even at low doses, the following SSRI medications have been used effectively to balance serotonin:

Prozac (fluoxetine)	Zoloft (sertraline)
Paxil (paroxetine)	Luvox (fluvoxamine)
Celexa (citalopram)	Lexapro (escitalopram)
Viibryd (vilazodone)	Trintellix (vortioxetine)

2. NOREPINEPHRINE

All too often problems associated with norepinephrine are not correctly diagnosed simply because doctors do not connect the physical symptoms, anxiety, and other disorders, with an imbalance of norepinephrine.

Symptoms of norepinephrine imbalance include:

- Lack of energy
- Lack of focus, concentration and organization
- Physical symptoms (such as chronic, recurring pain)
- Symptoms associated with anxiety (such as insomnia, panic, palpitations, elevation of pulse and blood pressure, etc.)

- Food cravings
- Weight gain with poor metabolism

In more than half the cases of a serotonin imbalance, there is also an imbalance of norepinephrine. But since most doctors do not know this, they are likely to treat physical symptoms with pain medications such as narcotics, muscle relaxants, and anti-inflammatories. Anxiety symptoms, on the other hand, are usually treated through tranquilizers, sleeping pills, and so on. These are short-term solutions at best—and in worst-case examples can result in dependency—but they do not resolve the problem.

SNRI: Serotonin and Norepinephrine Reuptake Inhibitors. These medications prevent neurons from reabsorbing both serotonin and norepinephrine at the same time, hence I refer to them as "dual action" medications.

The most commonly prescribed SNRIs are:

Effexor XR (venlafaxine ER)
Cymbalta (duloxetine)
Pristiq (desvenlafaxine)
Fetzima (levomilnacipran)

We have been working with these medications long enough to know that SSRI medications tend to reach a point of diminishing returns—that is, they are not as effective after a few months of taking them as they were at first. When this happens, most doctors will increase the dose of the medication to try to recover the early results. There is a better response though to the "poop-out" factor of SSRIs, and that is using diminishing or lack of effectiveness as a diagnostic tool. If SSRIs are not doing the job, then we have a clear indication that we have to look into balancing other chemicals alongside serotonin.

Now, as a class of mood normalizing agents, SSRI medications have a thirty- to thirty-five-percent remission rate (as remission is currently defined), which is good, but not good enough. The remission rate for SNRI medications goes up to about forty-five percent, which is better, but it means that more than half the patients who use it do not achieve full remission. When treating a patient, however, I choose the one agent that offers the greatest possibility of achieving results, and SNRI medications are often the ideal first-line agents. The best approach is to refuse to settle for minimal improvement and strive instead for one hundred percent resolution of all the underlying symptoms.

The sad truth is that the majority of patients who suffer with depression and anxiety disorders also experience a variety of physical pains and symptoms that are obstacles to achieving full remission. The physical symptoms usually disappear though when each neurochemical imbalance is addressed. So when pain and anxiety are among the list of symptoms, the first neurochemical that should come to mind is norepinephrine, with GABA second.

3. Dopamine

Dopamine is often lost in the shadow of serotonin, but it is often the most important neurochemical to balance when it comes to quality of life issues. There will be patients who will never enjoy full remission if dopamine is not addressed.

I find it useful to simplistically distinguish between *daytime*- and *nighttime*-related symptoms of dopamine imbalance to decide which medications to use. I have chosen this simplistic way to distinguish these symptoms. The "daytime" symptoms are more consistent with unipolar depression (though also possibly bipolar depression), while the "nighttime" symptoms are more related to bipolar mania or hypomania, or "treatment-resistant" depression and anxiety or more difficult-to-treat unipolar disorder. I will clarify these terms later in this book. Daytime dopamine imbalance symptoms include:

- Lack of energy
- Lack of motivation
- Lack of focus and concentration
- Decreased metabolism with weight gain
- Decreased sex drive
- Decreased drive in general
- Decreased memory
- Decreased executive functioning (performing intellectual tasks)

Symptoms associated with the imbalance of dopamine during the nighttime (which also affects someone during the daytime) include:

- Insomnia
- Racing thoughts
- Persistent and recurring anxiety
- Persistent and recurring depression
- Nightmares
- Agitation/restlessness
- Recurring pain (imbalances of norepinephrine and GABA more often than serotonin or dopamine, though they may also be involved at some level, can also cause recurring pain)
- Any other symptoms that would potentially worsen while attempting to sleep or relax (anxiety symptoms usually worsen when one is at rest, and obviously one is mostly at rest, or at least attempting to, during the sleeping hours.)

Dopamine is the brain's pleasure chemical—the "sex, drugs, and rock and roll" neurochemical. People with a dopamine imbalance are frequently those who try to self-medicate through behaviors or habits that produce momentary feelings of happiness such as illegal drugs, alcohol, smoking, sex, eating, and other pleasurable activities. Some patients are able to control these behaviors, but others get trapped in addictive or unhealthy activities. People who find themselves drawn to or abusing cocaine, amphetamines (speed in whatever form), diet pills, caffeine, energy/power drinks, sugar during the daytime, alcohol, cigarettes, tranquilizers, marijuana, and carbohydrates in the evening should definitely consider having their dopamine balanced.

When dopamine is brought back into a proper balance, patients have described their change of mood as "Getting their *mojo* back," "Becoming their old self again," and "Getting back into the game." What they experience is a resurgence of motivation, energy, and improved metabolism with the resultant weight loss, sex drive, and ambition they had enjoyed prior to the imbalance.

Wellbutrin XL (bupropion XL) is most often effective in addressing "daytime" dopamine imbalances with their related symptoms. As I mentioned earlier, Wellbutrin in almost every case works best when used in combination with other mood normalizing medications. "Nighttime" dopamine imbalances and their related symptoms are best addressed with the class of medications known as the "atypical" antipsychotics. These include Seroquel (quetiapine), Abilify (aripiprazole), Geodon (ziprasidone), Zyprexa (olanzapine), Risperdal (risperidone), Invega (paliperidone), Saphris (asenapine), Latuda (lurasidone), Rexulti (brexpiprazole), Vraylar (cariprazine), Caplyta (lumateperone), Lybalvi (olanzapine and samidorphan), Fanapt (iloperidone), and possibly more on the way. Remember, I have prescribed a lot of these medications and usually don't prescribe them for "psychosis." Since dopamine can be a bit difficult to balance, I've had many patients take both Wellbutrin and an "atypical" in order to balance dopamine both day and night, which when properly done means balancing dopamine 24/7. It needs to be turned on appropriately and off appropriately each day. Though dopamine can be the most challenging neurochemical to treat, it is the most fun, because when it is balanced, it restores the luster, vitality, and joy to a person's life.

4. GABA

GABA is probably the most under-appreciated and under-recognized neurochemical involved in mood disorders. Symptoms of GABA imbalance include:

- Anxiety
- Pain, especially headaches and neuropathic (nerve-related) pain, and pain in general
- Depression
- Low metabolism with weight gain
- Food, drug, and alcohol cravings
- Fatigue
- Poor focus, concentration, memory, and confidence
- Insomnia

Medications that are useful in addressing GABA are:

Topamax (topiramate)
Lyrica (pregabalin)
Neurontin (gabapentin)
Depakote (divalproex sodium)
Trileptal (oxcarbazepine)
Lamictal (lamotrigine)
Tegretol (carbamazepine)
Keppra (levetiracetam)

Lamictal doesn't actually affect GABA directly. It actually has actions that lead to inhibition of glutamate, which indirectly relates to GABA. Glutamate is the main excitatory neurochemical, while GABA is the main inhibitory neurochemical. This explains why enhancing the release of GABA and/or inhibiting the release of glutamate lead to calming, reduction of anxiety, reduction of somatic symptoms, improvement of sleep, reduction of depression and stabilization of mood. Lamictal is a unique antidepressant for treatment-resistant/bipolar depression, and is the only antidepressant that is also a mood stabilizer at the same time.

I list these medications as GABA-ergic for the sake of simplicity. The majority of them were originally anti-seizure medications. This label is misleading, since I prescribe a lot of them, often "off-label" for many reasons other than for seizure disorders, which I don't treat. These medications each have different mechanisms of action, but basically the end result is enhancement of GABA release and inhibition of glutamate release.

A Better Way to Do Things

How can doctors determine which medication or medications are going to do the best job in restoring the proper neurochemical balance? The approach I recommend is the unique approach I have learned and helped to create, a method of combining the right medications together in the right way, which is simple and innovative. I refer to this as the rational polypharmacy approach. The goal is to balance different neurochemicals at the same time, in the most rational and complete way.

I begin by prescribing a medication that should resolve the patient's primary symptoms Then, after a couple of weeks, and based on the patient's response and any remaining symptoms, I may add a low dose of another medication, and continue then to add, delete, and adjust the medications until every symptom and neurochemical has been accounted for and we have achieved *full remission* (the patient is fully well). We continue a follow-up program to ensure that the patient's brain is able to maintain normal mood functions. This can be challenging because the body's chemistry is affected by the ongoing development of the aging process and certain illnesses or conditions that are picked up along the way. Nevertheless, reaching full remission is achievable for most patients if we persist, and that is my goal.

The symptoms associated with each neuro-chemical are generalizations, and there are other chemicals and factors involved. Doctors need to be alert to the variations among individuals. For example, some serotonin symptoms maybe caused by an imbalance of dopamine, and vice versa. Some symptoms that sound like they are related to an imbalance of norepinephrine may actually be due to an imbalance of GABA. Being aware of how different people respond to different medications gives us a better understanding of the pieces to the neurological puzzle and serves as a roadmap to guide our diagnosis and treatment plan. Medications introduced into a person's system must be customized for that individual, because the neurochemistry of every individual is unique—that is, their own unique neurological fingerprint. The role of mood normalizing medications is to restore the normal state of balance in *this particular person's* nervous system.

As with any medical procedure, the more experience doctors have treating a particular condition, the more likely they are to develop an intuition about what medications to prescribe. The symptom-based approach I have described here is not only "patient-centered," but also allows doctors an opportunity to enhance their learning curve as they discover the benefits of the various medications.

Unfortunately, few doctors have learned the rational basis for choosing specific medications to treat specific problems. Therefore, they choose one medication at random, assuming that all SSRI's are basically the same and any success they might see is a matter of chance. However, these assumptions are wrong.

Cooking Up Wellness

Imagine the neurochemicals in your brain to be a sophisticated and complex chemical *stew*. Your doctor, then, is the chef who adds and stirs ingredients to produce the perfect recipe. When full remission is achieved, let the stew simmer. This is our strategy for maintaining the individual's improved health for the rest of his or her life. I may add spices and other ingredients to optimize the person's well being rather than settling for just good enough. I refer to this as the "fine zone," which is likely not complete remission. Once the recipe is just so, the end result can be a culinary sight to behold.

Chapter Five

"I'm Not a Pill Person"

She arrived at our office for her first visit with a grocery bag. In the examination room she emptied the contents of her bag onto the treatment table, and out spilled a variety of bottles filled with vitamins, minerals and herbs. I was amazed and amused at the quantity and diversity of natural supplements scattered in front of us: Shark fin cartilage, blue-green algae, MSM, colon-cleansers, and an assortment of organic remedies and health enhancing products.

She informed me that she was taking something like a hundred different capsules, drops, and scoops of powder every day and confidently asserted that they helped her cope with her various physical problems. Then she cautioned me that I should not try to prescribe any *drugs* for her, because, as she said, "I'm not a pill person."

I feigned innocence and asked why someone who is not a pill person was taking such a huge number of pills that sat on the treatment table. "Oh," she replied, "those are not the kind of pills I'm talking about, they're just vitamins and herbs, and they're all natural. These are the only pills I take because they're good for me." In other words, she was opposed to taking synthetic drugs concocted in a laboratory by a mad scientist in order to poison our society by mind control, sold by a greedy and evil pharmaceutical company, and in the long run would do more harm than good. Before she had even entered my office, she had me pegged for a "pill pusher," so she wanted to be clear from the start that she did not need any of my concoctions.

Assured that I fully understood her, we sat together and she produced a list of her physical problems, which started to unfold several times and nearly reached the floor. I remember having that uneasy feeling that comes over doctors when they are behind schedule, hoping for a quick visit, and realize that they will be planted in the exam room for a while. With all the willpower in me, I sat for the five to ten minutes it took her to complete the list. During that time she kept looking up at me to know whether I was still listening, so I maintained eye contact while taking notes and mentally strategizing how I would avoid falling further behind with my appointments.

Looking back on that visit, I now understand her surprise at the fact that I did not interrupt or try to rush her. As a matter of fact, I was doing my best to mask my anxiety because I surmised by the way she scrutinized me that she was used to having doctors react to her with impatience and a lack of empathy. When she pulled a stack of test results from her purse, she divulged her frustration, because several other doctors had told her all of her tests indicated she was in the normal range on all counts and there was nothing wrong with her. She was convinced that they had concluded she was a hypochondriac and showed her little interest, thoughtfulness, or concern.

After assuring her that I cared and would do my best to address her complaints, I said, "By the way, you do realize, don't you, every one of these items on the exam table are *drugs*? So what you have told me is that you prefer one type of drug over another."

She was, of course, skeptical and gave me a sideways glance as if to say, "I can't see where you're going with this, but I can guess that you are pulling some kind of trick." I then asked her if it would be okay for me to explain what I meant about different types of drugs. When she gave me a slight nod, I went on. The supplements that you are taking now to maintain your health are supposedly better than what I recommend, because they come straight from the earth. There are, however, a few risks with those supplements that you should know, just in case you have not read the fine print.

"First, it is possible to overdose on vitamins. For example, having too much of the B-complex can result in toxicity. Too much Vitamin B1 can cause heart palpitations, high blood-pressure, and insomnia; too much B2 can cause nausea, anemia, fatigue, and the list goes on. This is not just with regard to the use of vitamins, but I am also referring to herbs, supplements, and other 'natural' products that make promises without proof.

"Second, most of these supplements are not subject to any rigorous controls that ensure quality or that ensure that there is a standard amount of herb or mineral in every pill. For instance, if you buy a plant extract such as St. John's wort, one batch may contain more of the active ingredient and another batch may contain less. You never know exactly how much you are getting, which can be scary because there are side effects associated with St. John's Wort. These include dizziness, anxiety, headaches and sexual dysfunction.

"Third, even though the label on the bottle describes the beneficial effects of the product, there has never been any proof that the claims are true, and that is why the small print says: *statement has not been evaluated by the FDA. This product is not intended to diagnose, treat, cure or prevent any disease.* In other words, your type of drugs have not been monitored in their production, approved by any recognized authorizing board, and they admit that there is no evidence they can do what they claim.

"Fourth, merely because something comes from a plant or from the ground does not mean its health value is greater or more pure than something that comes from a lab. For example, some plants and weeds are poisonous and even deadly. In laboratory settings, these can be made to be very clean and pure with measured results and quality control.

"The *drugs* that I prescribe are safe for almost everyone when taken as directed. They are well tolerated overall and manufactured under strict controls. Their benefits and side effects have been carefully studied and proven before they are ever released to the public. In fact, for a medication to pass the government approval process, it has to be tested and retested until the strict rules of the FDA are completely satisfied of its health benefits and the limitations of its side effects." I want to make it clear, however, that it is not the FDA or bureaucrats to thank for the high quality and safety of medications, but rather the scientists/doctors that evaluate the products who are most qualified to ensure our safety and the pharmaceutical companies that provide the highest quality medications. Involvement by the government actually leads to the exact opposite. "Well," she said, "I'm just not a pill person. I believe in a holistic approach to good health." "That's great!" I replied, "Then I have the perfect thing for you."

I finally piqued her interest. I was then able to explain that the medications I prescribed are the most *holistic* products available because they do not introduce any chemicals to the body that are not already there. Instead, my drugs have no other purpose than to balance the body's resident chemicals so that it can heal itself *naturally.* I also pointed out the important distinction I make between the terms mood *altering* drugs, which I do not recommend, and mood *normalizing* drugs that target abnormalities in the nervous system that cause it to be imbalanced, and this brings the nervous system back into balance and helps the body to heal itself. This is true holistic medicine. She again nodded her head with only a little more enthusiasm and said, "Okay, then, I'll try them."

I now had to make up for lost time, so I told her there were a few things I had to do and asked if she had the time to wait for me as I attended to some urgent matters. She assured me she was in no rush and she would be there when I returned. I was able to see two other patients that did not require more than ten minutes each and went back to my office and scanned the charts on my desk to see if anything needed my immediate attention. I passed several tasks off to my staff and asked them to let other patients know I was running about a half hour or so behind. They were also to make certain that none of them were "flight risks" and were willing to wait.

Afterwards, I grabbed some samples, took a deep breath and returned to the examination room. She had been intrigued by the comparison of her drugs and my drugs, but I had her full attention when I announced, "Your other doctors were wrong. You are not a hypochondriac and your symptoms are real." I then explained that chemical imbalances would account for the various physical symptoms she had suffered. She admitted that my diagnosis made sense because for some time she suspected something in her body was out of balance. I assured her that I knew how to bring it back into balance using tested and approved medications.

In this woman's case, I could not see any reason to subject her to more testing because she had already undergone a battery of probes, blood panels and x-rays. I therefore looked over her test results to make certain nothing was missing and gave her samples of Effexor XR. We started with a low dose, and I explained that how she responded to it in the next couple of weeks would either confirm my diagnosis or lead us in another direction, but that we were going to beat this thing. Before leaving the office, I had her schedule another appointment two weeks out.

She was a different person when she returned to the office. She confessed that she was genuinely surprised that the medication was working and she was amazed at how much better she felt. I told her, however, that we had won a battle, but we wanted to win the war. When she first came to see me, she had that long list of symptoms and now most of them were resolved. I explained, however, that my goal was to address any residual symptoms as well, and that we were going to add a low dose of Wellbutrin XL to the Effexor XR and see if that would help clear up anything or everything that remained.

Within a month of her first visit, this feisty patient was in full remission and chose to get rid of her grocery bag of supplements. She decided they were no longer necessary because she was much better. There had been a point in her life when she lost hope that she would ever feel normal again. Today, however, she is still enjoying good health and understands that she never again has to feel as miserable as she did before we met. She remains a loyal patient and a great spokesperson, because several new patients were added to our practice in response to her referrals.

From Impatience to Good Patients

We both had learned important lessons in working together. Ideally, every doctor-patient relationship would be mutually rewarding and both parties would look forward to their visits. This is ideal, however it is seldom the same as reality, and every doctor knows there are patients who present significant challenges. I am usually up for the challenge, but I refuse to let it become a battle of wills. Instead, I see it as a puzzle to solve, and if I can be creative enough, I will find a solution that works for both of us. When I convince patients that what they have been doing is taking them in the opposite direction of their goals, get them to turn around, and together watch them get better, I have the deeply satisfying reward of knowing that I have changed a life for the better. So, to tell the truth, I enjoy those patients that pose a challenge and generally grow to love and appreciate them. Helping them to improve their mental and physical health encourages and assures me that I can certainly help the patients who are cooperative and therefore easier to treat.

Changing Lives and Improving Attitudes

Some of the troublesome patients doctors see are not inherently annoying, but they have been programmed to be wary when they visit our offices. This is because they are frustrated with the government's "strictly business" attitude toward medical care, the conflicting advice of numerous health care professionals, and having trudged through "HMO nightmares." In other words, the imperfections and glaring abuses of the entire system have ruined the doctor-patient relationship for many people.

Sometimes it is in the office of the family physician where negative attitudes are formed between doctors and patients. The sorts of problems that arise tend to fuel themselves. For example, if after a few visits the doctor begins to suspect that the patient is malingering (exaggerating or faking symptoms to get out of work or receive compensation, which happens all too frequently) or is suffering from a condition that is known to be caused by stress, or if the person appears to be a hypochondriac, the doctor will reveal his condescending attitude toward that person. Many times the doctor does this unconsciously.

We do it with body language, the roll of our eyes when the receptionist tells us that the patient is on the phone for us, and with the tone in our voice when speaking to them (we talk to them as if they were five or six years old). The whole office staff will then adopt this same attitude, and sensing it, the patient will feel minimized and possibly resentful.

Unfortunately, many doctors do not know how to most effectively treat stress-related conditions, such as TMJ and fibromyalgia, preventatively, or how to address stress when it intensifies other symptoms. Doctors, nurses, and therapists sometimes conclude that they are dealing with a neurotic or obsessive person and assume if they would simply "chill," and do the normal routine of diet and exercise, their symptoms would go away. Then there are the *cheats* who use their doctors to try to get time off work or pain-relievers or other medications that they will abuse. Therefore, doctors and their staff are conditioned to make judgments about certain people. When they guess wrong about a patient who cannot reduce their stress because of a chemical imbalance, the results are sometimes tragic and can even be deadly.

The patient-doctor relationship can either be a bridge we use to connect with each other for the benefit of the patient's health, or it can be a hole we dig together and get stuck in so that neither one of us goes anywhere in regard to improved health. If a patient has been mistreated by another doctor and staff they will likely be prepared for rejection by the time they enter our office. If we respond like all the other doctors (and the behavior and attitude of some patients practically begs us to do so) then they will experience yet one more failure at the hands of the medical community. When we judge them for being noncompliant or challenging, we merely dig the trench deeper. Life lesson: If you find yourself in a hole, stop digging.

Doctors can interrupt and put an end to the negative cycle through the remarkable power of genuine care. This means that the interest a doctor shows in the patient must be positive, sincere, understanding, and kind. When the patients who need the healing assistance of mood-normalizing medications receive this sort of attention, they soon become more cooperative and are less likely to be as desperate and needy as when we first began to treat them.

Transforming the Doctor-Patient Relationship

Patients, like the grocery-bag lady, that at first seem to be obstinate, have become receptive to my suggestions when I simply take the time to establish rapport, show concern for their well-being, and explain myself with clear and easy-to-understand instructions. A primary goal I have with *every* patient is to get to know him or her as a person. In fact, I *need* this kind of personal knowledge in order to "feel" my way to an approximate diagnosis as to what sort of chemical imbalance we will have to treat. A personal knowledge of the patient not only helps guide my diagnosis, but it also enables us to enjoy more effective communication during subsequent visits.

For the same reason, in most instances, I diligently apply myself to educating my patients regarding the neurobiology of their chemical imbalance and how the medication I prescribe will address it, much like I am doing in this book. I will draw (admittedly cheesy) illustrations, provide statistics, use analogies (like the "light switch" in an earlier chapter), and give them examples so they can understand what we are trying to achieve and how we are going about it. In this way, we can maximize their cooperation in the healing process and minimize their worries or resistance. Most patients are fascinated to learn even a fraction of information about what goes on inside their brains and how mind and body function in tandem.

There are some people, however, that do not want any education from someone like me, a licensed member of the same system that has already abused them and made their lives difficult. Frequently, these are also the people who do not want to hear that their suffering is quite literally caused by something in their head. As far as they are concerned, their head is fine. In terms of being intelligent and bright thinkers, they usually are. It is their body that is in pain.

I have learned to be diplomatic with these patients. I may not tell them that what I am prescribing is a mood-normalizing medication to resolve the chemical imbalance in their brain. Instead, after listening to their symptoms, taking a family history and examining the area that is the primary focus of their concern, I explain that it is pretty clear to me that they are suffering from either chronic inflammation of some sort, or I may give a medical label that is recognizable such as Fibromyalgia, Irritable Bowel Syndrome, or other "diagnoses" to reassure them it is a real disorder. I may then prescribe, for example, Effexor XR (venlafaxine ER), without necessarily telling them that it works to help their own neurochemicals do the job they were intended to. Since some are not interested in receiving an education from me, I let them know that if my diagnosis is correct they should be feeling the benefits within one to two weeks. I have learned to begin this treatment even with patients who do not have signs or symptoms of any mood disorders if the symptoms they do present with are most consistent with stress-related problems.

If patients are feeling better within that short time, which they will be if my diagnosis is correct, and ask me about how Effexor XR works, I merely explain that its intended use is to improve mood and reduce stress, including its physical as well as its emotional manifestations. Since they already understand and appreciate the difference they have experienced, they become more willing to at least consider the possibility they may have a chemical imbalance that affects the mood and physical body at the same time.

Note to Doctors Who Want a Thriving Practice

Simply being a "good doctor" by treating patients as people rather than cases or symptoms will result in solid referrals. Good communication skills and listening skills are crucial in order to practice this type of medicine. Other family members who have suffered from anxiety, depression, bipolar disorders, and other manifestations of neurochemical imbalances, such as chronic pain disorders, chronic insomnia, fatigue, etc., that have most likely gone misdiagnosed or undiagnosed, will literally rush to the office to ask if it's possible to do the same thing for them that I did for their brother, daughter, aunt or whoever else in the family may have been afflicted with it. It is important to understand the crucial role that genetics plays with regard to this subject. There is no more effective way of getting word-of-mouth referrals than by enthusiastic people who are eager to tell everyone about how wonderful life has become for them since seeing me.

I no longer see patients like the grocery-bag lady as difficult, but rather as the sort of people that I can help the most. I cannot describe what it feels like to give hope to people who are hopeless and who have settled into despair and watch them light up. By changing my attitude towards them, they have responded in kind and changed their attitude towards me. Whether you are doctor or patient, you can appreciate how much smoother and more enjoyable the healing process can be when there is a cooperative relationship of mutual respect. A meaningful and rewarding relationship in which the patient feels at peace in trusting the doctor, and the doctor is aware of that trust, is a rewarding relationship indeed. More and more, the ideal has the potential to become real.

The Value of Holistic Medicine

Some of my patients are surprised to discover that I am an holistic doctor. They did not expect a physician embedded in the Western medical community to buy into and practice holistic healing. However, knowing that the central nervous system does not exist separate from the body nor does the body exist apart from the central nervous system, I appreciate how everything works together—one system, organ, appendage, supplying the needs of the others. There is no getting around the fact that thinking affects mood, mood affects organ function, organ function affects the immune system, the immune system affects mental and physical response to stress, stress affects thinking, and so on.

In treating mood disorders, I do not discourage my patients from seeking psychological counseling, massage therapy, acupuncture, nutrition, aerobic and anaerobic (such as yoga) exercise, and having a spiritually centered life, *so long as they also appreciate the necessary work we do together in balancing their chemicals.* I stress my role in the holistic process. Apart from having a proper chemical balance, other treatments are often not going to produce what I refer to as a *true cure*. In fact, no other treatment is going to resolve the patient's condition if there is a significant chemical imbalance that is not corrected. The body's chemistry is where healing *begins*. Once the neurochemicals are functioning as they should, then the patient has the necessary foundation for making progress through counseling, diet, and other forms of therapy.

I am dogmatic about using only holistic medications to produce the correct neurochemical balance. Holistic medications, to some people, sounds like a contradiction. Mood normalizing medications, however, are holistic because all they do is assist the body's natural functions in normal response to stimuli and provide service to other neurons and parts of the body. In this way, I play my part in holistic treatment to achieve what I term a *true cure*, by helping the body to heal itself.

Having said this, I do try to warn my patients about certain products that are advertised as *holistic*, but can actually introduce something into their bodies that works against their healing or can even be harmful. A patient who takes unnecessary supplements or an excessive amount of any particular supplement, can produce toxicity that actually poisons the body. This class would include supplements like St. John's Wart, 5-HTP, SAM-E, GABA, and others. I have seen patients who take capsules, powders or pills that are manufactured in uncontrolled environments—resulting in varying degrees of chemicals from dose to dose—or use these so-called natural remedies without proper medical supervision, and can suffer serious mental disorientation and confusion.

One patient in particular comes to mind. He was brought to my office by his wife because she said he was suffering from dementia and she wanted to know if it was the onset of Alzheimer's disease. The first thing we did was discontinue the supplements he was purchasing through the mail that were supposed to improve his memory, and within forty-eight hours he regained his normal and—in his case—brilliant mind.

A treatment is, in my opinion, not holistic unless it works with the body's natural chemistry in order to bring the mind and body together. Mood normalizing medications function in exactly this way, by balancing neurochemicals already present in the nervous system and thereby engaging the whole body in the healing process. The results are not only a healthier physical and mental life, but also greater cooperation in the mind-body functions necessary for good health.

HEALING
— THE —
MIND AND BODY
VOLUME 1
SECOND EDITION

— SECTION III —

THE STATE OF MEDICINE AND HOW IT IS AFFECTING THE MIND AND BODY OF THE PATIENT

- JOURNEY OF DISCOVERY
- UNCOVERING THE COVER-UP
- TAKING THE "PSYCHO" OUT OF PSYCHOSOMATIC
- WHAT YOUR DOCTOR SHOULD KNOW (BUT MAY BE AFRAID TO ASK)

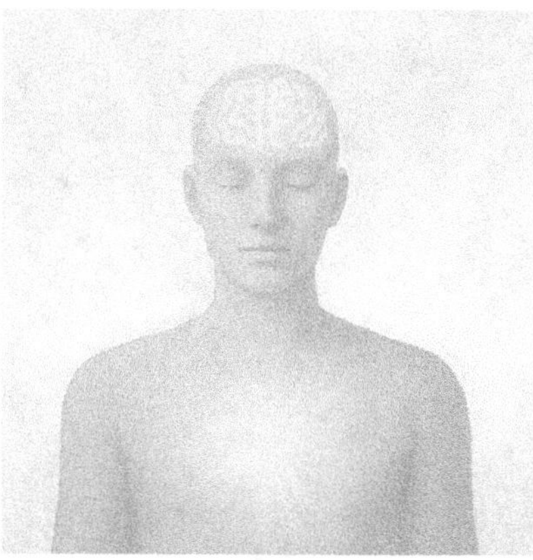

PAUL D. CORONA, M.D.

CHAPTER SIX

JOURNEY OF DISCOVERY

This chapter will involve us in some time traveling. You are going to move with me through my initial experiences in the practice of medicine, to my questions and concerns, through a season of putting new medications to good use, and then coming to a series of breakthrough insights which will bring us to the present. Along the way you will learn something about me, but more importantly, you will learn the background of what has become the most effective way of treating mood disorders while also addressing a host of physical complaints. I will reveal to you how I came to develop The Corona Protocol, after practicing and researching in the office for quite a number of years learning how to treat patients most completely and effectively.

The journey began well over twenty-five years ago. Family Medicine was an easy choice for me. I have always had a deep interest in people and have been fascinated by the variety of personality types, cultures, temperaments, and behaviors. My medical career has given me the opportunity to engage with families in the full spectrum from pediatrics to geriatrics. Walking into the examination room is always exciting for me, because I never know what awaits me within. I do know that by teaming up with my patients to discover what lies at the root of their complaints helps us to work together to make life-enhancing decisions. The face-to-face interaction with my patients has always been my favorite part of practicing medicine.

Even though I was a premedical student at the University of Southern California (USC), the "Introduction to Psychology" class was one of my favorites. As a Biology major and an aspiring doctor, it was natural for me to also study Psychiatry and neuroscience (the study of the human brain and nervous system). I didn't think I wanted to practice Psychiatry full-time. I chose Family Practice since it combined Internal Medicine (adults) with Pediatrics, Gynecology and Psychiatry all at the same time, which was perfect for me since I was interested in all those aspects of health. These subjects continued to pique my interest all through med school and into my residency. At that point, the interest became a passion to study and understand human behavior.

While a resident at a big and busy Southern California hospital, I worked in what are known as "locked wards," where at-risk patients (those who are out of touch with reality or could pose a potential threat to themselves or others) are closely monitored and hopefully stabilized. In these two units, I came into contact with patients suffering from Schizophrenia and severe Bipolar Disorder for the very first time. I wondered how one could become so disturbed that one could no longer function in society. The question I kept asking was how a brain could be altered drastically enough to produce these kinds of tragic illnesses. From that point forward, I determined that I would find out.

There was something a physician said during my residency that grabbed my attention. According to his estimation, in more than fifty percent of the patients that doctors treat, the underlying problem is *psychosomatic*. I have found this estimate to be true in the over two decades of my practice, and if anything, the estimate is too conservative.

Seeing that so many of my patients suffered from psychosomatic conditions, I became intensely interested in how the nervous system could affect physical health. I found that it was necessary to look into my patients' psychological makeup as well as their physical symptoms in order to ensure that the treatment I recommended would be effective.

When the first SSRI (Serotonin Reuptake Inhibitor, an antidepressant) was introduced in the mid-1980s (Prozac), I quickly familiarized myself with its uses and effectiveness in a clinical practice. Prozac (fluoxetine) was a definite improvement on the medications available to physicians prior to its release. Even though I saw some encouraging and even dramatic results, a number of patients experienced unpleasant and unwanted side effects, and for many, incomplete results. It made some other patients worse. Prozac provided doctors with a significant treatment for depression, but it was certainly far from perfect.

For a while, Prozac became a favorite target in the media, but the negative press it received was riddled with errors and misconceptions. Even today some patients express apprehension because of rumors they heard or a talk show they watched that sensationalized a tragedy that had to do with the misuse of Prozac and other factors, and was in actuality, not a result of the medication itself. The most important result of Prozac entering the market was that it made very clear the role that neurochemistry plays in depression and that serotonin is definitely a factor in mood disorders.

The next medication to reach the market was Zoloft (sertraline), which was also an excellent product in its time. It was gentler than Prozac and better tolerated by some. This is because Prozac is more "potent." Zoloft soon became a popular choice for mood disorders, and rightly so.

A third SSRI, Paxil (paroxetine), came out in the late 80's to early 90's (during my residency program). Paxil tends to produce a *calming* effect in most patients, unlike the *activation* many people experience with Prozac and Zoloft. Paxil found a niche among people with anxiety and depressive problems by exploiting the fatigue-related side effect to some patients' advantage. For that same reason it sapped patients' energy. It made waking in the morning a struggle and was difficult to discontinue using. I found that I prescribed it less often than other medications.

The real hero today in the field of antidepressants is Effexor (venlafaxine), and when it proved to be very potent, my interest in antidepressants surged. Effexor was the first modern antidepressant that balanced not only serotonin, but also norepinephrine. Initially there were problems with Effexor, because patients had to take it twice-a-day and in some cases it produced nausea (its competitors referred to it as side-Effexor). Therefore those of us who prescribed antidepressants preferred the SSRI class that had been released earlier because they seemed to produce fewer side effects.

The Really Big Breakthrough

By far, the most important stage of my journey of discovery occurred with the arrival of Effexor XR (the XR on the label means "extended release"), which my patients would be able to take only once-a-day. Soon after I began prescribing it, patients were raving about it, asking questions like, "Doc, what the hell did you give me?" I would ask them how it differed from the other medications they had tried, and their response could be summed up in the words of one patient who said, "Let me count the ways." They had more energy, better focus, improved sleep, lost weight, and some of them reported that they had relief from headaches and other chronic pain conditions that had plagued them for years.

Some of these people had bounced from doctor to doctor, and had been treated by everyone from orthopedic surgeons to neurologists to rheumatologists to cardiologists, gastroenterologists, pain specialists to chiropractors, to "holistic healers" to health food stores, and the list goes on. You get the idea. They had been x-rayed, poked and prodded, had multiple tests and other diagnostic studies. They had been operated on, given physical therapy, injected and swallowed a variety of medications without experiencing anything close to the positive results that Effexor XR (venlafaxine ER) produced.

Since those early encounters with the remarkable performance of Effexor XR, I have heard reports from patients who have explained the benefits of this remarkable medication in regard to a number of different complaints. Various aches and pains diminished and disappeared, high blood pressure dropped to healthier levels, symptoms associated with acid reflux, fibromyalgia, and irritable bowel syndrome (IBS) diminished or resolved. I have also seen incidences of infections, asthma and allergies decrease. Some of the "mystery" symptoms for which doctors had not been able to find a cause simply vanished. Although my previous experiences with SSRIs familiarized me with the way an imbalance of serotonin could affect patients, I had never seen the kinds of problems resolving as quickly or as well as what I was witnessing by balancing serotonin and norepinephrine at the same time with Effexor XR.

A few striking stories from patients stand out in my mind. For example, one patient, who was preparing for a third surgery, had suffered for several years from chronic sciatica and lower back pain. The surgeon was reluctant to perform the same surgery, but the patient begged him to do it, because the previous surgeries had provided him at least a few months of relief. I informed him of some of the results other patients had been enjoying with Effexor XR and provided him with samples I had in the office. A couple of weeks later, he called to tell me his pain had vanished. His surgeon, even though happy that he did not have to perform the operation, could not understand how this medication resolved his pain.

One day the patient arrived at my office with his most recent MRI. "Dr. Paul," he said, "Look at these areas on the MRI with the discs slipped out of place and all the scar tissue." He wanted me to understand it was a structural problem, and not his imagination, causing the pain. When he asked for an explanation, I surmised the medication was working on the nerve that traveled through that area of his back and helped to balance from within the nerve that had to travel through that mess. Once the nerve was working properly, even with the swelling and surrounding scar tissue, and the disk pressing against it, the result was the pain in the sciatic nerve resolving. That was the best explanation I could come up with at the time, and it appears I was right. I also explained to him that the pain made him anxious. His anxiety, in turn, caused additional pain, which may have contributed to what had become a vicious cycle. Today, this grateful patient needs nothing more than an occasional over-the-counter anti-inflammatory.

Another patient suffered a very unfortunate case of chronic vertigo for almost 30 years. In spite of the multiple workups and MRIs, the specialists who worked her case, and a variety of medications, nothing effectively corrected the problem. Eventually she found her way to my office.

Like the other physicians—I am assuming—that she had previously visited, I began with an examination of her ears and sinuses, because sensitive mechanisms for keeping our balance are located in the inner ear and there are a number of conditions that cause disturbances in the inner ear. However, after checking for something that could affect her physical condition, I was unable to find any obvious source of vertigo. This was not surprising for me, because physical examinations do not always pinpoint causes for the symptoms she described.

While trying to determine a diagnosis, I noticed during her first visit that she almost always seemed to be anxious. In one of our appointments, I brought this to her attention and explained that a chemical imbalance can sometimes affect the nerves in the inner ear and that could be the cause of her vertigo. She agreed to take Effexor XR for a few weeks to see if it could help. Within days, however, we were both amazed to see her condition resolve. Though she has occasional mild and brief spells of vertigo today, it is nothing like the chronic and severe problem that she suffered for many years before taking Effexor XR.

One other woman was suffering with chronic recurring yeast infections, and had gone to specialists who had tried several different creams and pills to no avail. Since starting Effexor XR, she hasn't had one for several months.

I have lost count of the number of patients who have experienced relief or resolve of a number of physical, stress-related symptoms. If anxiety persists for any length of time, sooner or later it will compromise a person's immune system. As a result, the normal infections and intrusion of foreign bacteria that our bodies fight off every day begin to overwhelm our defenses. Once we address and reduce the anxiety, the immune system returns to normal function and a host of symptoms can disappear within a relatively short period of time.

The Missing Link

As I witnessed the rapid and remarkable improvement of more and more patients, I found myself wondering why other doctors were not noticing and publishing the same results. None of the medical journals were reporting on these sorts of phenomena, none of the seminars or lectures I attended addressed the issue, and no other doctors ever mentioned it. Even today the majority of physicians do not appreciate or do not attend to the chemical link between the mind and body. The potential gains of treating every patient as a whole—neurology, physiology, cardiology, orthopedics, and even psychology and spirituality—are far too great to be ignored. Since no one else was talking about these breakthrough cures, I decided that I would start telling other people about it—doctors, patients, nurses, and anyone else willing to listen. After all, helping the brain to heal the body, and reconditioning the brain through the body, is the *missing link* in medicine today. The real *missing link* is the mind-body connection. These conditions, primarily caused by neurochemical imbalances, are treatable and curable by the breakthrough method that I have practiced and developed to achieve such excellent results.

THE NEXT STAGE OF THE JOURNEY

The diagnosis and treatment of mood disorders and all the symptoms that result from them would be much easier if we could determine exactly which neurotransmitter was not doing its job and treat it with a designer medication made to assist that specific chemical. We have not yet advanced our science that far, although we have made significant improvement in determining which chemicals may be imbalanced. Another difficulty is that it is rarely only one neurochemical causing the problem, so even if one medication resolves some of the symptoms, it will not help with symptoms caused by another neurochemical, which brings us to my next major breakthrough in the treatment of mood disorders.

THE SELECTIVE COMBINING OF MEDICATIONS

Suppose a doctor was seeing a patient whose initial complaints had to do with such things as fatigue, constant muscle soreness, and irregular sleep patterns, which after an interview and thorough physical examination, we traced back to depression as the cause. Since, in most cases of depression, serotonin is the primary suspect and norepinephrine is usually an unrecognized second one that imbalances, and due to the fact that I have had significant success in treating both emotional and physical complaints with a dual-action agent, I had found back then that Effexor XR (venlafaxine ER) or the second dual-action agent Cymbalta (duloxetine) were the best, while most doctors then and now prescribe an SSRI (medication that only balances serotonin). My most standard approach was trying Effexor XR and comparing it to Cymbalta before the follow-up appointment set for two weeks later.

When the patient returns, there is a noticeable difference. First, he may tell the doctor about changes he has noticed. He knows though that he is not completely better, and even though the medication has helped some, he still has all the same symptoms. Then he begins to describe the minor side effects of the medication. That doctor may then respond to his report by explaining that we still need more time to see what the medication can do and that the side effects he described are not serious and will continue to diminish.

However, if the patient is then referred to me, I am concerned that he has not experienced greater relief and I notice also that he is very fidgety. So I ask, "Are you nervous?" To which he responds, "Why do you ask?"

ME: Well, it seems like you can't hold still. The whole time you've been in the exam room you seem nervous.

HIM: Yeah, I guess I am sort of nervous.

ME: Is there anything in particular that's making you anxious?

HIM: I guess, now that I think about it, I am worried about the fact that I feel a bit better with this medication and don't feel as well as when I stop it. Now you want to switch to a different one? I don't want to be addicted. Does this really mean I am suffering with something that's just mental?

There are many reasons for me to be concerned by what he has said, but at the same time, there is nothing unusual with what he is thinking.

So I tell him that even if he is depressed, it is not "just mental," but is physical and can be treated. Then I explain to him that it is now pretty obvious that a serotonin malfunction is not the only problem. There are three or more neurochemicals that play important roles in maintaining a normal and well-balanced mood. Then, depending on the ongoing symptoms he describes and my observations, I may prescribe another medication to take with the Effexor XR or Cymbalta (and more currently Pristiq or Fetzima), explaining my reasons for doing so. Again, I give him samples and send him on his way with instructions to return in another two weeks.

Why am I seeing this patient at two-week intervals? The medications I have prescribed do not immediately produce the chemical changes we hope to see, especially at low doses, which are my preference at the start. The effect of the medications are cumulative, so it generally takes a week or two to determine whether they are going to do the job, though some patients report radical differences almost overnight.

The next time I see the patient, he is a changed man. He is smiling when I enter the exam room, and shows no symptoms of anxiety. In fact, even if he did not tell me he felt better, I could see in his posture, skin tone, eyes, and other features that his sleeping was improved, his energy increased, and he had a better outlook on life. As soon as he opens his mouth, he is thanking me, telling me I am a miracle-worker. He then goes on to tell me how his life is significantly different, that he is happier and more creative than he can remember in years, and he is now back on track. "How'd you do it, Doc?"

In the thousands of instances of treating patients with mood disorders, this story is an accurate description of what I see all the time—in fact, it is what I see in the majority of my patients using The Corona Protocol. We understand the human brain so well, and I have seen it respond to the right combination of the best available medications so that I am not at all surprised when patients enthusiastically report a radical improvement in their mental and physical health. In the cases that show only moderate improvement, we continue to tweak the medications, adding or subtracting those that are most or least effective, until we achieve the optimum results which is always the goal when using The Corona Protocol effectively. Fortunately, we live in a time when new and improved medications are being tested and released all the time.

There are a number of reliable indicators to determine if a patient requires a combination of medications to resolve their symptoms. I have discovered that balancing norepinephrine with serotonin can, in many cases, resolve physical complaints and anxiety-related symptoms, such as insomnia, panic attacks, and agitation.

Resolving Stress

Antidepressant can be a misleading term when talking about the use of medications for balancing neurochemicals in the brain. The complexity of the brain's anatomy, the communication back and forth from the various regions of the brain, how it responds chemically and electrically to *everything you experience in your environment as well as within your body*, how its own thoughts affect it, and its links to every part of your body, means that reducing the benefits of a breakthrough mood-normalizing medication or "antidepressant," results in the assumption that it is only for people who are depressed and undervalues its other positive effects in people who are not depressed.

On occasion, patients have asked me if their stress is what causes their symptoms or if the symptoms are the cause of their stress. If it were only that simple! Both stress and stress-related symptoms work against each other, perpetuating and often increasing the intensity of the negative effects of the other. That is beside the point, because we do not have to answer that psychological *chicken or the egg* question, because we now have medications that address both stress and symptoms at the same time. It's both the mind and the body. It's both the chicken *and* the egg.

Amazing Results

The next big question for me to tackle was why the medical community had not embraced Effexor XR (venlafaxine ER) as I had. Certainly other doctors must have been seeing the same results that I had observed with my patients. I could not be the only person watching people transform before my eyes. What I came to learn is that other doctors were not using Effexor XR the same way I had learned to administer it, and were obviously not looking for what I was seeing.

When Effexor XR was first launched, the manufacturer notified doctors that it would balance three neurotransmitters according to the following scale: *Serotonin* at low doses, *Norepinephrine* when prescribed in mid to higher range doses, and *Dopamine* at the highest recommended dosage. The logic of feeling good is simple. If the proper function of one neurochemical improves a patient's general feeling of well being, then that feeling is increased if two neurochemicals are working within the norm, and so on. So, like most other doctors who wanted to see the medication working at its maximum effectiveness, I prescribed Effexor XR at the higher range of dosages by starting low and tapering up quickly, as the company recommended. At first it seemed that the high doses worked well for many patients, but it soon became clear that there were troubles in paradise. At the higher levels, the wonder drug produced nausea, increased activation, fatigue, dry mouth, sweating, insomnia, weight gain, and elevation in blood pressure for some patients.

My frustration with Effexor XR was that within two weeks most patients reported feeling really good, but with an increased dosage, the side effects began to appear and create discomfort. I decided not to give up on Effexor XR, but to keep the dosage in the lower range. Immediately my patients and I were thrilled with the results. Patients enjoyed positive changes quickly at the lowest dose and many continued to report the best results with only a slight increase in the dosage by the second week, but still keeping the dose in the lower range. This was a ground-breaking discovery for me and became a defining moment in my career.

The most important highlight of this new development was the fact that at the doses I was prescribing for my patients, Effexor XR was not supposed to produce a significant change in norepinephrine, yet it obviously did affect that neurochemical as well as serotonin. Many of my patients who had been using some other SSRI (medication that only balances serotonin) switched to Effexor XR at low doses and found the anxiety as well as a number of physical symptoms that had not been affected by the earlier medication began to resolve.

Unfortunately, most doctors, even to this day, who prescribe Effexor XR still believe what they were told by the manufacturer and are convinced that to achieve the desired response from norepinephrine that they have to prescribe the higher doses. They usually taper it up to 150 mg, and it is commonly believed that 225-300 mg is the optimal dose. I have rather found that 75 mg is the most common optimal dose with 37.5 mg the second most common best dose, with 150 mg third, 225 mg fourth and 300 mg fifth. This truth about lower often being better has not been the conventional thinking with regard to not only Effexor XR first, but also all of the psychotropic medications.

Several years ago, I learned that I wrote more prescriptions for Effexor XR first, then Pristiq (desvenlafaxine) second, in the nation, and that I write the most prescriptions for antidepressants and mood stabilizers in general, at least for a family doctor. I was not pleased to receive that news, but rather saddened, because it means that other doctors have not taken full advantage of the newest and best medications, and their prejudice prevents them from providing their patients the greatest improvement possible with improved health and relief from oppressive mood disorders.

Another Wonder Drug

A third significant event in my journey of discovery was learning how to prescribe Wellbutrin. As I mentioned above, one of the draw-backs of Effexor XR is that it produces unwanted side effects at higher doses. Unfortunately, however, there are some people whose condition requires something more than what they get with low doses of only Effexor XR. I refused to accept the idea that we had to negotiate a trade between feeling good and putting up with unpleasant side effects. So I began to combine low doses of Effexor XR with low to mid-range doses of Wellbutrin XL (bupropion XL) knowing that it targets dopamine, with a minor effect on norepinephrine.

Since an imbalance of dopamine results in fatigue, depression, decreased motivation, apathy, anhedonia (loss of interest and pleasure), decreased memory, decreased sex drive and sexual functioning, and decreased focus, I discovered that patients not only experienced a more significant response from the two medications, but that the Wellbutrin also eliminated some of the unwanted side effects of Effexor XR.

Doctors have at times augmented (or combined) SSRI medications with Wellbutrin, but the effects are not as significant as combining it with Effexor XR. Since this combination provides the best ratio of simultaneously balancing serotonin, norepinephrine, and dopamine, it has proven to be a very effective treatment for most patients who suffer from unipolar disorder (depression and anxiety) as well as certain variations of bipolar disorder. Because of the proven effectiveness of Effexor XR and Wellbutrin, I have administered them to patients with mood disorders and chronic physical complaints with excellent results.

I have not heard of any other doctor combining these two medications and have not read about it. One reason other doctors have not discovered the power of this *dynamic duo* is because few realize the importance of norepinephrine in mood enhancement and physical symptoms that are emotionally generated, while balancing dopamine leads to an improved quality of life for many.

A second reason is because many doctors think of Wellbutrin as an alternative first-line choice of medications. In reality, only rarely should Wellbutrin be used as a stand-alone medication, because it is primarily an *augmenting agent* (agent that is added to the previous agent). It just happens to be the best augmenting agent on the planet. Since many doctors are not aware of differences that occur when balancing three neurochemicals rather than two, they have not reached the ultimate goal of optimum health for their patients.

A Fortuitous Conference

Having attended many conferences for speaker training (having been hired by several pharmaceutical companies to lecture to doctors), I can assure you that the majority of them are neither interesting nor informative. I have learned to use them as a good excuse to get out of town and enjoy a restful weekend. The speaker-training program I attended in Chicago several years ago was different and became a fourth major revelation in my journey.

Soon after the opening remarks, I found myself intrigued with the subject being addressed and began taking notes as fast as I could write, struggling to keep up with what I was hearing. Afterward, I was motivated to make use of what I had learned and began rewriting my notes and organizing them on the plane ride home. Those notes proved to be very valuable and became the basis of many of my writings on bipolar disorder.

I had attended the conference because I had discovered that I needed to be able to present to patients and others a reasonable and meaningful explanation about a medication called Zyprexa (olanzapine). Although the normal use of this medication is to serve as an antipsychotic, I had found it to be effective in the treatment of bipolar disorder and I needed to be able to explain why it worked in this unorthodox usage. At that time, I had considerable experience with this particular class of agents and had worked with Haldol (briefly) and Risperdal (risperidone) for years in treating the more difficult cases of eating disorders and difficult "treatment-resistant" depression and anxiety disorders. What I took home from the conference was the realization that many hard-to-treat patients were actually suffering from bipolar disorder. The fact is, I had been treating a large number of cases of bipolar disorder through the years, but I had not known what to call them.

This information taught me to include a class of medications referred to as *"Atypicals"* (atypical antipsychotic medications) and use them in combination with Wellbutrin for the challenging cases of bipolar disorder that is so common in a primary care setting, though it has usually gone unrecognized. Some doctors are concerned that the use of Wellbutrin in treating these patients will "activate" and "destabilize" them. This, however, is rarely the case when the process is approached carefully and the patient's progress is monitored. If, however, Wellbutrin does produce activation, then the dose of the atypical (mood stabilizer) can be increased to balance it. Conversely, if the atypical dose causes fatigue when it reaches its most effective dose, it is generally resolved with the addition of Wellbutrin.

When most doctors think of bipolar disorder, they have in mind the most extreme version, Bipolar 1, which affects only one-percent of the population. In most cases, bipolar disorders are subtle, difficult to detect, and are often mistaken for "treatment-resistant" depression/anxiety disorders, adult ADD, or chronic insomnia. What has opened up the field of more powerful treatments, however, for addressing these disorders is the combination of medications I have been describing. I love discussing this subject with doctors, because they are typically amazed when the light turns on and they realize that bipolar disorders are so commonly seen in the office and are so easily and effectively treatable.

GABA AND TOPAMAX

The most recent major event in my journey of discovery has been through my recognition of the importance of the chemical GABA (gamma amino-butyric acid) and what occurs in the body and mind when it is imbalanced. I had previously focused on the other three neurochemicals more than GABA, but I have begun to appreciate the importance of having it in balance as well as the others. Remember, GABA is the main inhibitory neurochemical, and glutamate is the main excitatory neurochemical.

I knew about GABA/glutamate imbalances (and chemicals related to it hence what I term GABAergic), because I had worked with medications such as Neurontin (gabapentin) and Depakote (divalproex sodium), which were originally designed as anti-seizure medications. Over the years they have mostly been used "off-label" for relieving headaches, pain prevention, and as anti-anxiety agents. I have also come to appreciate the important role that Lamictal (lamotrigine) plays in treating patients with bipolar depression. Lyrica is related, and may be helpful for pain and anxiety prevention. The medications in this "anti-seizure" class are very helpful for bipolar depression, treatment-resistant depression and anxiety, reducing somatic complaints, mood stability in general and other benefits. When patients have not responded well or have had only partially positive results with a regimen attempting to balance serotonin, norepinephrine and dopamine at the same time, or whichever of these three need balancing, GABA and glutamate had been the last class of medications that I really started to appreciate more over time. Among this class of medications, however, the one that stands in the winner's circle is Topamax.

Topamax (topiramate) has been used effectively in the treatment of chronic headaches and various nerve-related pains. What I have learned, however, is that Topamax has decent mood-stabilizing properties and is excellent for helping patients lose weight safely and effectively. It's rare in this field of medicine to have a mood-stabilizer with positive effects on depression that causes weight loss. In addition to Wellbutrin XL and stimulants, these are the only psychotropic medications that lead to weight loss. Most of the others can cause weight gain while some are weight neutral. That's one of the reasons that topiramate is such an incredible medication with huge potential. Unfortunately, it is under-prescribed and these conditions are under-treated.

However, the potential problem with Topamax can be cognitive side effects for some, such as difficulty in putting thought into words. This potential effect subsides, however, as soon as treatment ends and is not a major issue for most patients who benefit from it as long as the dose is not increased too high for that individual.

In summary, I more commonly start with an SNRI (Pristiq most commonly in recent years), with an SSRI more often a second-line agent. I often augment with Wellbutrin XL, an atypical and/or a GABAergic agent, in the correct combination for that individual. However, when patients have not responded well to a treatment that is designed to balance serotonin, norepinephrine, and dopamine, I have learned to target GABA as well, and generally with satisfactory results. In this way, I came to see that GABA and glutamate had been the last missing piece of the puzzle.

The Journey Never Ends

Giving patients hope makes an enormous difference in their treatment, because humans are not merely their bodies, they are souls who think, dream, desire, and feel. Because I can give them hope, patients rarely resist an innovation in their health care so long as I take the time to explain to them why it is likely to work for them. In fact, they are often eager to try something new, because many of them have seen several doctors and specialists without getting any better. They also appreciate my suggestions, because they can see in what I offer them my commitment to helping them get better. So, once I realized there was no other field of medicine that could help patients more dramatically, and in a relatively short period of time, than the The Corona Cocktails I have learned to mix together by hand-crafting in order to create a unique blend which best matches the individual in front of me. It has been an exciting journey of discovery, and it has been a fun ride to be a part of. I then decided to give up general medicine for the most part, though I mix my skills in Primary Care as well as Psychiatry in order to make the best decisions about treating both the body and the mind. I focus on the whole person at the same time when I treat Mind-Body disorders, understanding the connection between body, mind and spirit. I treat patients who have multiple physical and emotional complaints, and work with them until all of the problems are resolved, or at least as close as we can get. Full remission is always the goal of The Corona Protocol for every individual, and making this reality come true has become a passion that has guided my life.

From that introductory course in psychology at USC over 30 years ago to the discovery of the "missing link" of medicine and of life itself, my journey has been thrilling. It is gratifying to look back and reflect on how far I have come and how many people I have helped. At the same time, I never forget that the journey does not end. There will always be that next person who is suffering and needs the help of someone dedicated to their care, and there will always be that next breakthrough medication to introduce and tweak until we get the results we desire.

Chapter Seven

Uncovering the Cover-Up

We have come to a great mystery. If the new model of understanding medicine is the interplay between the mind and body, and if properly balancing neurochemicals in the brain is the key to repairing and optimizing the mind-body connection, and if we have powerful and effective medications that can be used in rational and creative combinations, then why are there so few doctors aware of these breakthroughs? Why are so many people still suffering needless mental and physical anguish? Why do we not hear more about the rising tide of improved health care? I doubt that you will like the answer when you hear the truth.

Quite frankly, there are powerful institutions in our society that are controlled by people who are less concerned about your health than they are their personal investments, interests, prestige, tradition, or influence. As I said before, given the remarkable improvements I was consistently seeing with my patients, I was baffled as to why other doctors were not talking about achieving these same results. As I sifted through medical journals and spoke with colleagues, I could not find one piece of information regarding what I had learned regarding the effects of the new medications when applied in such a way as to target specific neurochemicals.

The method I used to treat both mind and body is one that I developed through what I refer to as the "rational trial-and-error" approach. Pharmaceutical companies can recommend general dosages for patients, but they cannot establish one specific dose that will work equally well for everyone, so the doctor has to start somewhere and then do some adjusting. I've learned how to specifically tweak the medications, stop the medications, lower or raise the dose, add on another agent, and then do the same thing with each additional medication. In retrospect, I think of my research as a complex medical puzzle that is made of pieces from a variety of sources, and my job is to solve this living human puzzle sitting in front of me. Once all the pieces are put in place, they formed a clear picture of what I needed to learn to develop improved patient care in order to help patients and teach other doctors how to do it most effectively.

Along the way, however, I came across a number of obstacles that could have prevented me from pushing forward and has effectively stymied the progress of doctors and their patients. I cannot blame other practitioners and they have my sympathy, because I know how easy it is to be intimidated by institutions on which doctors must rely to keep their practices flourishing. Nevertheless, some of the institutions that are supposed to be looking out for the welfare of the patients are, in reality, taking steps that guarantee people will not receive the best possible care. The list of offenders, beginning with those that are most responsible for blocking the flow of information and advance of health care are as follows:

1. The FDA/The Feds and legal system
2. Insurance companies, especially managed care
3. Doctors, the field of Psychiatry, medical societies and the medical profession in general
4. Pharmaceutical companies
5. Patients themselves, and society in general

"WHY DOESN'T MY DOCTOR KNOW ABOUT THIS?"

As I explained in the previous chapter, most doctors still believe that Effexor XR (venlafaxine ER) does its best work at higher dosages. But as I discovered, this information is wrong. In actuality the very best results usually come from lower doses, and many people have better results from combining lower doses of Effexor XR with Wellbutrin XL (bupropion XL), while sometimes adding other medications and combining different medications together depending on the patient's condition and response to treatment. I have discovered that several different combinations of medications at varying doses, ranging from one to two to about four medications at one time are needed in some patients in order to achieve the best results. This depends on the severity of the patient's condition, with usually two to three medications for the average patient in order to get the best results. Despite the miraculous results, I have seen again and again that while using this method I have devised during 25 years of private practice, I have never read or heard of any other doctor doing the same thing or applying the same method in the same way that I do it.

One problem is that these medications were never marketed properly, and their best uses were never made public. This continued to be the case even after doctors had discovered that these medications could do more than what the manufacturer had indicated. In this instance, however, the fault lies not with the manufacturers, but rather with the FDA, which prohibits these companies from advertising or even talking about the medication's "off-label" uses (uses that they were not originally intended for). Using psychotropic medications "off-label" just happens to be the most cutting-edge way to use them. My method relies heavily on "off-label" use, which is why it works so well. In restricting the free speech of what the research and development labs of pharmaceutical companies have discovered about a medication, doctors are left to their own devices to discover the truth. Unfortunately, for one reason or another, most doctors never go beyond what is written in a brochure or what they are told by a sales rep. Even the content of the lectures is controlled by the FDA as to what can or cannot be said to doctors. They are very concerned that they *approve* all discussions and that they are "on-label" only.

Ignorance of the beneficial uses of medications is not the only problem. An example is that many people in the medical community are either misinformed or not well enough informed regarding all the facts pertaining to bipolar disorder or how it can be treated most effectively with "atypical" antipsychotics, as I mentioned before. Unipolar disorder is easier to treat, though most doctors don't even know how to treat this most common variation of neurochemical imbalances in the most effective way. When it comes to treatment of either bipolar disorder or unipolar disorder, pharmaceutical manufacturers recommend prescribing high doses of their products for maximum effectiveness, but those levels are usually unnecessary. These recommendations are very misleading because they are inadequate and because they fail to distinguish that most bipolar disorder is not the most severe type, referred to as Bipolar I, but rather consists of subtler variations of bipolar disorder, which are usually misdiagnosed or undiagnosed. These more subtle variations are much more common. At this point it would be wonderful if the government could intervene by requiring manufacturers to be more specific about different doses for different variations and by educating doctors to the many benefits of these medications for many different problems other than what they are advertised for, but that type of rational action would be against their very nature. Lower doses prove more effective in the vast majority of cases, but this message gets lost in the confusion. Doctors are left to figure all this out by themselves, and unfortunately most never do.

The correct methods of lower doses and combining medications together gets lost if one pays attention to standard medical information. Doctors wait for studies in order to change what they do, and, since rational polypharmacy is difficult to study in the "traditional" ways, doctors don't learn it and therefore don't do it. I have found the only good way to do this is by learning it through seeing a lot of patients over many years. I urge other doctors to learn how to do it in the same way.

FDA to the Rescue?

Why is the FDA unable to do anything to clear up the confusion, fix the problem, and speed up the process of getting the best medical care to the greatest number of people? The fact is, the FDA *is* capable of making huge strides in correcting the problem, but those in charge have chosen instead to compound it. With the exception of Bipolar I, the

FDA does not allow pharmaceutical manufacturers to freely study or even discuss other variations of bipolar disorders. Manufacturers are only allowed to promote their products strictly for Bipolar I and not the other variations. As a result, doctors receive filtered information and are left in the dark about the powerful tools at their fingertips that they don't know how to use. Consequently, what they encounter is only the negative side effects of high doses of the medication without ever even knowing about all of its benefits or appreciating that results that are better tolerated would be seen if they started the medications lower and tapered them up more slowly, and combined them together in the right way.

Obviously, if the FDA will not allow the pharmaceutical companies to research the variations of bipolarity since they control if and how the studies are carried out, then they certainly are not going to allow them to mention "off-label" uses of their medication in the treatment of those variations. However, this is precisely the information that doctors would find to be most helpful. Without it, they continue to write prescriptions according to the recommendations of the manufacturers. Many primary care doctors choose to not even see patients who have bipolar conditions, but refer them instead to a psychologist who can't prescribe psychotropic medications, who may go through years of therapy just to make a diagnosis, if at all. Psychotherapy can be invaluable for certain patients, but for most the addition of the correct psychotropic medications often leads to the quickest and most complete results.

Sadly, the majority of patients who are recommended to a psychiatrist by their family physician will opt not to follow up or commit themselves to psychological counseling only, without considering medications that may be desperately needed. Patients may find it more difficult to get insurance coverage for counseling, and each therapy session is much more expensive than a visit to the family doctor. If a patient does take the big step to see a psychiatrist, they are then more likely to get the care they need in order to get the best long-term results. The problem I have seen though is that psychiatrists train primarily about the mind, but not very well about the body, so they often fail to understand how one affects the other so intimately. Therefore, most psychiatrists do not take a keen interest in their client's physical symptoms or appreciate the relevance of those symptoms in the diagnosis of the overall problem. Even if they do, they usually don't know how to resolve these physical symptoms most effectively.

There are also other pieces of information that psychiatrists typically miss: namely that the *low and slow* method of prescribing medications provides the most effective treatment with the best results that are best tolerated. Psychiatrists tend to push the medications to the higher dosages rather than combine lower dose medications. They also tend to prescribe a lot of "band-aids" (tranquilizers, sleeping pills, etc.) rather than focusing adequately on prevention (though other specialists and primary care doctors tend to do the same). Primary care doctors can most readily appreciate the slower and gentler medication approach. They understand this connection because of their general understanding of the physical body. They just need to appreciate how the mind/brain relates to it. Second, most psychiatrists and primary care doctors alike do not understand the full range of bipolar disorders as well as the many variations of unipolar disorders that require individualizing pharmacotherapy. This is usually best accomplished by combining psychotropic medications with different mechanisms of action together in a rational symbiotic way. This method is the best tried and proven way to achieve our treatment goal of full remission.

When a doctor follows the suggested directions for prescribing these medications, they inadvertently give the patient too much too soon, resulting in unwanted side effects. Because of their bad experiences, both doctor and patient may become disenchanted with these medications in the future and may resist trying them again. Manufacturers are shooting themselves in the foot, because their suggested levels work against the patient, and the result is that doctors are scared off and stop prescribing products patients cannot tolerate. When the next new product is launched, doctors may be apprehensive and may avoid using it right away, if at all. Patients often avoid trying something else if they have had a previous bad medication experience. The end result is that the patient loses.

Because of a dreadful lack of information, for which the FDA is responsible and that pharmaceutical manufacturers perpetuate (seeing that they have no choice), this inevitably hurts patients more than helps them. If they have any experience with medications, it turns out to create more problems than it resolves. So the next time a doctor says something like, "I want to put you on antidepressants for a few months," the patient may immediately respond, "No thanks, Doc. I've been on antidepressants before and they made me feel miserable. I just don't think they're for me."

The "Drug" Companies

Pharmaceutical companies have three primary goals: First, to make money for their shareholders and employees. The second is to get the FDA to approve their product. The third is to market their product to make it as impressive as possible in order to compete with other companies' products. The reality though is that the way these goals work out in legislation and the marketplace rarely works in the patient's best interest.

The FDA and manufacturers of pharmaceuticals do not advertise the fact that combining lower dose medications together rather than pushing any one medication to its limit (as manufacturers tend to promote their product over competitors) achieves the best results for mood disorders. This truth gets lost in the race for approvals, sales, and dollars. End result? The patient loses.

Different Agendas

The agenda of pharmaceutical manufacturers is in conflict with the agenda of the doctor in family practice as well as the psychiatrist. The manufacturers want their product to be approved by the FDA as quickly as possible and to appear as attractive as possible to doctors and consumers. If they can guarantee quick results at high doses, they are not above recommending elevated doses, even if the low-dose method is more effective in the long run. Pharmaceutical companies rush their studies and enhance them with partial information, which can be misleading.

Doctors are not in such a rush. They will be caring for a patient through the whole time that it takes for a treatment to work effectively. The doctor's work is for a lifetime. A doctor has to take time in order to evaluate the big picture, especially primary-care doctors. Quick results are not always the best results. A quick turnaround time for treating mood disorders is certainly desired, but is usually achievable with better results if done in the right way.

When a pharmaceutical company tests a new product, they have to *simulate* a situation as best they can, but they are rarely working with real-life circumstances. The people who participate as patients in these studies must have a *pure* form of the condition that is being studied without the complication of any other medical problems that could potentially skew the study. For this reason, there are many people who apply to be subjects for a study, but do not make the cut since they have other things going on with them.

Therefore, the results of *any* such study are questionable, because they do not reflect the true condition of an average patient. Doctors rarely see patients whose condition is *pure*. They see average patients that usually have multiple problems. That is why patients must repeatedly return to the doctor's office until their condition is resolved, because each time they visit there is some other aspect of their heath that requires attention.

I tend to read medical journals with a critical eye, because if the evidence is gathered in a way that is not true to life, then the results are not reliable. Most of the studies reported in medical journals have a narrow focus that will bias the results. Studying the mind-body connection in a lab or in a clinical trial holds little promise, and, as important as the test tube may be, it provides limited information about what works in practical application. In fact, there is no greater understanding of what people suffer, and what is most likely to promote healing, than years of hands-on experience with real people.

The Least Realistic Agenda

Pharmaceutical manufacturers behave poorly in part because the FDA forces them to think and act according to its agenda. They really have no choice but to play along if they wish to be allowed to survive. If they don't play the game, then they have no other choice but to lose against the FDA. To tether creative minds to bureaucrats, who are perhaps the most non-progressive thinkers in the medical field as well as in general, just doesn't work. This inefficient and uncaring system can and will bog down the most important and necessary research that is needed to keep a steady stream of better and safer medications flowing from labs to the general public.

Since the FDA mandates that pharmaceutical companies only mention the approved use of a medication, they will keep this information from doctors for fear of being intimidated, reprimanded, or fined by the government. For example, the label on Effexor XR says that it is an antidepressant and makes no mention of its effectiveness with anxiety, chronic recurring pain, and other physical symptoms that are stress-related as well as multiple other disorders it is helpful for. Doctors who play it safe by following the rules on the label may not be comfortable exploring off-label uses of a medication, and thereby deprive their patients of potential gains they would otherwise enjoy. Only after they read a journal article about the off-label benefits of this or that medicine, will the timid physician possibly take a step in the right direction, following a trail that others have blazed. For some patients though, by the time their doctor finally gets around to making the most of a medication, it is too little too late.

The FDA is the least qualified institution to make important decisions regarding the uses of medications. Only people who are qualified in the field of health care and medicine, and have experience in treating various conditions, should be making these decisions. Until that day arrives, the truth about the best "off-label" uses of medications will be hidden in mystery.

Who Can You Trust? Not These Sources!

I have found that the worst sources of medical information are:

- Family and friends (as well as others with little or no medical knowledge or training)
- The media (televised news, brief articles in magazines, etc.)
- Pharmacists
- The Internet—good medical information is hard to come by on-line. If it is not the FDA misinformation, it is usually some nut case or quack who is just plain wrong.

Imagine learning to play golf or learning how to ride a bicycle by doing nothing more than reading about it on the Internet. Who has ever become proficient working with computers just by reading the owner's manual? The same is true of medicine, because there are so many variables in dealing with the complex systems that function to maintain the body's equilibrium. Add to that challenge the questionable credibility of people who post articles on-line. Chat rooms are full of disgruntled people who have a bone to pick and want everyone to know their opinions, which are, for the most part, invalid. For example, the websites about Effexor XR and Pristiq (desvenlafaxine), which just happen to be among the best medications ever invented, are completely misleading and untrue. (This is also the case with every other psychotropic.) There are thirteen-year-olds who pose as adults or experts and, regardless of how precocious they may be, they are in no position to give sound medical advice. This also applies to any other people of whatever age that are not qualified to have medical opinions, much less advise others regarding medical issues.

If a pharmaceutical company decides to get approval for a medication's use, other than its original indications, the FDA requires them to spend a ludicrous sum of money and to jump through a maze of flaming hoops. Once again we have the government to thank for the inflated cost of the medications we need in order to maintain our physical and emotional health. If doctors were consulted and allowed to determine the uses of a medication based on what they have actually observed it do for patients, the costs would come way down and we would have a much more effective system of approval.

Again, if the role of the FDA is to protect consumers, doctors, and manufacturers they certainly are not doing a good job. Doctors, manufacturers, and even consumers could accomplish this more effectively at much less cost. Imagine consumers actually getting advice on medical issues from actual medical specialists, whose goal is that you achieve the best care and the best results you can. The effectiveness of an institution or community that is not politically driven is many times greater than a system that runs under the enormous weight of bureaucratic tomfoolery, waste, greed, and corruption. The fact that this subject is critical to the health of countless patients is the very reason the FDA should not be involved. Given the glaring inefficiency of our federal government in regard to the educational system, utilities, industrial out-sourcing, and anything else in which it is involved in the public domain, do you think this same institution should be making critical medical decisions for you and your family?

Watching the Feds regulate medicine has angered me for years. The reality is that patients' and doctors' decision-making is controlled by an institution that is least qualified to make those decisions. Lawyers unfortunately run medicine, not doctors. Nonetheless, like many doctors, I have felt powerless against this almighty system. Sometimes I feel like a lone voice crying in the wilderness, and this is why I felt the need to write about this subject. We have put up with too much and suffered for too long, and it is time to do something to fix it.

THE FDA: THE ENDLESS PURSUIT OF FAME AND FORTUNE

I have often wondered, "What is the big deal about the "off-label" use of medications? Why is the government so threatened by this? Don't they realize this is just how doctors do things? Don't they realize this is the best way to practice medicine that benefits patients the most?" Even if they did know something about the practice of medicine, it would not matter. Our government is not as concerned about our health as it is with power, posing, and most of all, making money.

Our government often acts like the playground bully that scares other kids into handing over their lunch money. This particular bully sees pharmaceutical companies as easy targets with deep pockets. The government is tough and greedy, and the manufacturers are pretty much defenseless. No wonder manufacturers are paranoid. The government can enter their offices at any time and investigate whether they have ever advocated the off-label uses of their products. The government is currently receiving hundreds of millions upon multiple billions of dollars through retroactive fines, as well as other forms of creative extortion that they have come up with, levied against manufacturers. The way our government sees it, the money is there for the taking, so they take it in order to be able to grow and keep on growing. If it were up to the government, it would never shrink. Therefore, it has to be forced to. The reality is that it is bloated and desperately needs to lose some weight.

Pharmaceutical companies are not the bad guys. In fact, every family in America and millions around the world can be thankful for the money and labor they pour into the development of new and better products. It's a small price to pay for the cost charged compared to the results that are seen. Consumers at the pharmacy counter tend to blame these companies for their greed, when actually it is the government who deserves our disgust. We are the ones who pay the cost of government approval and fines imposed on manufacturers. The power and reach of the FDA was already rapidly growing under President Clinton's administration and those prior to him, but its growth had been exponential during the so-called "conservative" Bush administration. It is not surprising then that during the current Obama administration that the FDA as well as all branches of government have metastasized at a dizzying rate. Thanks to the outcome of the 2016 election, at least now we have real hope. The price at this point of producing a pharmaceutical product from concept to release has grown to an obscene rate, and these costs are passed on to the patient, who is the biggest loser of all in this shameful mess.

Malpractice: We All Lose (Except the Lawyers)

Because of the increase in malpractice lawsuits, doctors retreat further and further every year into the practice of "defensive medicine." If a patient is not suing them (many times for an error no greater than what any human makes every day), they are paying hefty fees for insurance to protect their families and homes. Who bears the weight of their insurance premiums? The patient. And who suffers for the conservative approach they take to health care and their reticence to go out on a limb on behalf of people who need something different than what they get from everyone else in the medical industry? The patient.

For centuries, the practice of law was considered one of the three "learned professions," which meant it was an honorable pursuit that required an advanced education and a commitment to a high ethical standard. For that reason, law firms considered it unethical to advertise their services, even in the telephone directory. In fact, some states had laws on their books that prohibited lawyers from advertising. Within my lifetime there has been a dramatic change in the marketing and advertising of law firms—obviously, seeing that you cannot drive through an inner city or watch television without seeing the faces of a number of attorneys plastered everywhere. In a 1977 Supreme Court ruling, lawyers were given the right to advertise based on the first amendment, and they have certainly taken advantage of this.

Guards have had to be briefed and posted at airports whenever an airliner crashes and passengers are killed. The guards are responsible to protect the surviving families from attorneys who will immediately hit the airport with their business cards in hand. The ambulance chasing (personal injury) attorneys are the only ones to consistently profit from the sort of litigation that terrifies pharmaceutical companies and doctors, as well as any perceived "deep pockets." Their feeding frenzy around the medical community with frivolous lawsuits continues to drive up the mounting costs of health care. By encouraging lawsuits, they seduce people into believing they have a chance to "hit the lottery," which arouses the greed of the average person since pharmaceutical manufacturers and doctors are viewed as having "deep pockets" which are ripe for the picking.

Keep in mind, however, that their pockets are not nearly as deep as are the pockets of the bureaucracy. In the end, all of our pockets get picked, and it is the lawyers and government that hit the lottery. The legal system when it comes to this subject is quite simply out-of-control. Lawyers and the government win and consumers lose, as usual. (I don't mean to offend or disparage all attorneys, just some.)

I Rest My Case

The following are examples of FDA meddling that have caused irreparable damage to the general public:

1. The Vioxx/Bextra scam

These anti-inflammatory products had a decreased risk of bleeding ulcers and stomach irritation in general compared to standard anti- anti-inflammatories. They should never have been taken off the market, yet we were led to believe that the FDA did this to protect us. Doctors learned that there was a very slight risk that these medications could promote congestive heart failure when given to elderly patients. By merely being armed with this information we would naturally be careful in prescribing them. Aside from the risk, that could easily be managed, the benefits of these medications were invaluable. The FDA, however, was not interested in the benefit of the medications and made a nonsensical decision that has left millions of patients to suffer needlessly.

2. THE ESTROGEN SCARE

Another concern that has been overplayed in the media has to do with risks associated with women who are given female hormones as treatment for various physical problems. Because of the panic that was generated by the bad press, many women either discontinued taking estrogen and other hormone supplements or refused to take them when they were recommended. Again, there were more women who benefited from estrogen treatment than there were who experienced complications from it. Experts in the medical industry quickly learned the potential risks and also learned to adjust treatment to avoid those risks. In fact, the more serious problems occurred for those who had taken estrogen supplements without proper medical supervision. Otherwise, most women enjoy significant benefits from estrogen treatment at low to moderate doses if it is taken for at least three to five years beginning at the onset of menopause. I would refer you to the research and work by the late Dr. Dan Mishell at USC and other reliable sources about the role of hormone replacement. A number of women would enjoy its benefits well before menopause and there are others who could use extended treatment afterwards.

What is required to increase the benefits and reduce the risks is the *ideal* practice of medicine in which decisions are based on such things as the patient's family history, current physical condition, and rational discussions with their doctors. In this ideal situation, the physician is able to communicate the facts that are relevant to the patient's condition and how to best proceed. The patient and doctor stand in the best possible place to consider the patient's case and be able to make sound decisions in order to achieve the best results for each individual. No one outside of the patient-doctor relationship should be making these decisions for them. Certainly no one should be allowed to frighten or intimidate either the patient or the doctor into deciding for or against a particular strategy to address the patient's health care. Sketchy science about "bioidentical" hormones stepped in and took advantage of the needless concern that was spread. They have duped many people into believing that their hormone replacements are superior to the more scientifically proven hormone supplements. This is yet another case of good press combined with bad science, and the unfortunate result was that the truth was lost in the madness.

3. The So-Called "Black Box"

For patients and doctors, this is perhaps the most damaging and nonsensical action taken by the Food and Drug Administration (FDA) to date. In 2004, the FDA issued a press release that began:

> *The FDA today issued a Public Health Advisory announcing a multi-pronged*

> *strategy to warn the public about the increased risk of suicidal thoughts and behavior ("suicidality") in children and adolescents being treated with antidepressant medications.*
>
> *The agency is directing manufacturers to add a "black box" warning to the health professional labeling of all antidepressant medications to describe this risk and emphasize the need for close monitoring of patients started on these medications. The FDA has also determined that a Patient Medication Guide (MedGuide), which will be given to patients receiving the drugs to advise them of the risk and precautions that can be taken, is appropriate, and is in the process of developing one.*

The "black box" is the most severe warning that the FDA can apply to a medication and it prohibits manufacturers from advertising reminders to doctors of the product's availability. The FDA also requires manufacturers to provide a "Patient Medical Guide" (circumventing the patient-doctor relationship) that describes the risks of giving antidepressants to children, adolescents and young adults up to the age of 25, and for what uses the medication has been approved or not approved for them. We might wonder what clinical studies were performed, what statistical research was gathered, and what experts in the medical field were consulted to move the FDA to such dramatic action. The answer, however, is "none of the above," rather they made this decision based on the findings of their own advisory committee, "as well as what many members of the public have told us." The actual information that the FDA had in hand indicated that suicide was related only to Prozac (fluoxetine), though I doubt this finding. In fact, in studies conducted with "five selective serotonin reuptake inhibitors (SSRIs) (Celexa, Prozac, Luvox, Paxil and Zoloft) and four 'atypical' antidepressants (Wellbutrin, Remeron, Serzone and Effexor XR)," there was "no reported case of a suicide."

Prozac (fluoxetine) has been targeted for years since it was released, because it had become the one antidepressant best known to the media. For a few weeks, Prozac enjoyed celebrity status, making the rounds of talk shows and being blasted by television and newspaper reporters and Scientologists. Statistical evidence, however, clearly shows that suicide rates have decreased since Prozac came out. The sad cases of parents whose teenage children took their lives were used to sensationalize the negative possibilities that were attributed to Prozac and other antidepressants. If there is one thing I have learned about the media when it comes to creating public panic regarding medications, it is that to sensationalize usually means telling sensational lies.

I grieve for the parents who have lost children to suicide—or any other cause of death. I understand the despair of suicide and how difficult it is for anyone in the depressive person's relational network, whether family or friend, to always be able to understand or provide help to that person. The association of antidepressants to increased risk of suicide is sheer nonsense. The truth is that it is actually the other way around. When the press created the furor that led to the FDA's actions, I predicted that the warning and new restrictions would themselves lead to an increased number of suicides. Sadly, my prediction proved to be accurate.

The fact that people suffering depression should consider suicide comes as no surprise. A normal, healthy mind does not find comfort in thoughts of self-destruction. Suicide is a risk even when depression is treated, but it is a far greater risk when not treated properly. Therefore interviews among depressed children, whether prior to or after being weaned off of medication, will naturally indicate that they have thoughts of suicide. So the results of FDA interviews reveal nothing more than what simple logic would tell us, and certainly do not prove that antidepressants are at fault.

In some reported incidents of suicide among teenagers who were prescribed antidepressants, the suicides occurred after they discontinued use of the medication, often by taking themselves off of the medication *cold turkey*. A doctor would usually not advise a patient to instantly stop taking an antidepressant, because doing so can result in disorientation and disturbance, or worse yet, a quick recurrence of depression, anxiety, or mania. If there were other cases of teens who committed suicide while on an antidepressant, they would need to be examined one by one to ascertain exactly what went wrong, and whether they stopped taking the medication without their parents' knowledge. This decision may have been initiated by the parents themselves because of fear based on misinformation. The recommendations of doctors working with parents and family members should be the primary focus, since these parties together are likely to make the best decisions without interference from outside sources.

The government paints with a large brush that easily paints over the needs of individuals. The harsh reality is that the government doesn't care about you. In the particular instance of the "Black Box" warning being issued, the government's ill-conceived actions cost pharmaceutical manufacturers millions of dollars in the recall of their samples to provide the new warning on package inserts, which are useless pieces of misinformation that doctors and patients shouldn't be reading anyway. The cost has been, of course, passed on to the consumer. When the actions of the FDA were publicized, some people were so alarmed that they stopped taking their meds, parents stopped providing antidepressants to their children, and doctors avoided prescribing antidepressants for fear of being sued. The total cost of the FDA's irresponsible actions in terms of loss to the Pharmaceutical industry (which then negatively affects the consumer), decreased health care due to physicians' worry about malpractice risk, increased expense to the patient, and unnecessary deaths, has yet to be calculated. If it were, you would no doubt be justifiably angry.

Why the FDA Should Not Make These Decisions

Research scientists and other experts in the medical community were outraged by the FDA's unilateral actions and the fact that the government did not bother to first consult with them. There are subtleties involved in assessing the value of an antidepressant that the FDA advisory board either did not consider or, more probably, did not know. The major research and information they relied on did not distinguish bipolar disorders from unipolar anxiety and depressive disorders. If most doctors find it difficult to make that distinction, how could the FDA possibly do so, and on the wide scale that such research would require? That miscalculation has tragically led to the unnecessary deaths of many by suicide.

The fact is there is a slight risk when patients with bipolar disorder are given medications that are designed to target depression, since they could quickly jump from depression (the *downside* of bipolarity) to mania (the *upside*), which could result in suicidal thinking. As far as I know, and I carefully looked into it, this concern was never addressed by the FDA. Nevertheless, this subtle, yet vital, distinction could dramatically affect any research on the effects of antidepressants and how the results of that research would be interpreted.

Like most government institutions, the FDA is politically and economically driven and is much less concerned with scientific scrutiny than with getting the next year's budget that they desire. Therefore, the FDA is susceptible to corruption and decision-making that is based on poor quality information. For example, a parent's testimony before Congress regarding a teenager who committed suicide while on medication will influence the FDA's response more than the facts provided by experts that have the most bearing on antidepressants. The decisions and actions that follow will promote an attractive media image for the FDA, because it will look like they are actually doing something on the public's behalf. Their heroic image, however, will continue to be undermined by the dark reality of the continuing number of deaths for which they are responsible.

Frequently we hear about medications that are being used in Europe and Asia to effectively treat patients who have conditions that are still very daunting to American physicians. The problem is that when a company decides to introduce these medications to the United States, they are instantly thrown into a tangle of useless committees, being pushed from one committee to the next for "further review." We are supposed to believe that the reason these medications are held up in the sticky web of bureaucracy, while people are dying, is because the FDA is busy protecting us. In most of these cases the FDA is doing the American citizen way more harm than good.

Insurance Companies: Unmanageable "Managed Care"

I am going to state the fact as simply and clearly as possible: Insurance companies have little concern for patients or the truth. I know that sounds harsh, and I don't mean to generalize since thats not always the case. However, they are among the wealthiest corporations in the world and for them the bottom line is dollars, not health or quality of life.

"Formulary" coverage for medications is one of the fundamental flaws of managed care. "Formulary" refers to the medications that insurance companies agree to cover and those that they will not cover. These determinations are made regarding all medications, but they especially impact mood-normalizing medications. When doctors prescribe medications that are not within the company's formulary, they must submit paperwork to justify their decisions, and that report goes to the company and their committees for a final decision. Of course, patients rarely even know that this behind-the-scenes correspondence is going on, but assume they are receiving the best treatment their doctor can provide. I wonder how horrified they would be to discover the truth.

Doctors do not appreciate being dragged away from what they should be doing—namely, treating patients—in order to go off and do paperwork or EMR (electronic medical records) or any other inefficient system that wastes valuable time. I dictate all of my notes and try to limit paperwork to a minimum.

Under the managed-care system, doctors are not free to make decisions they have been trained to make and are in the best position to make on behalf of the patient. To keep life simple and spend more time in the examination room rather than behind their desks, doctors will opt for the generic substitute of a medication, which is almost always the cheapest and lowest-quality product available. In the long run, not only are the patients receiving less help than what is available to them, but doctors are being deprived of the education that they would gain through experience with better products.

Every company that provides insurance for its employees is aware of the radical jumps in the cost of health insurance policies over the last ten to fifteen years. Therefore, companies are constantly shopping the least costly premiums on the market. Small companies are practically forced into HMO insurance policies. Most of the low-cost coverage provided by managed care does not include "psychiatric" services.

Here are examples of the expected results:

- Doctors do not want to provide services for which they will not be reimbursed.

- Patients are hesitant to mention potential psychiatric problems if it will increase their insurance rates or make it more difficult for them to qualify for insurance for now or the future. Doctors realize the unfair cost to their patients if they bring up the issue of psychological needs, so they may try to protect them by saying and doing nothing about those needs.

- Insurance companies which are heavily involved in managed care (i.e., HMO's) often require patients with mood disorders to see a psychiatrist in order to qualify for coverage for prescription medication to address the disorder.

- A visit to a psychiatrist or psychologist may or may not be covered by an insurance company. Generally, if coverage is provided it is extremely limited in terms of the psychiatrist one may see and how many visits are allowed.

- These plans tend not to attract the highest quality psychiatrists, who tend to spend even less time than other psychiatrists with patients that aren't involved in these plans.

- A psychiatrist may not prescribe medications to a patient who they know will come for only one visit. The psychiatrist will have to interview the patient on follow-up visits to determine if they have the correct medication and dosage. Even when the medication is working, the psychiatrist may want to address the mood disorder from the standpoint of the patient's psychological make up, and this could require many visits. So, simply stepping into the door of the psychiatric office for the first time could entail many more visits which the patients may not be able to afford and the insurance company will not cover.

- Another reason is when primary care physicians have to refer patients to a psychiatrist, they do not gain the much-needed experience of treating mood disorders, even though they stand in the best position to treat the vast majority of patients.

- Patients may be hesitant to see a psychiatrist because of the stigma that is still attached to seeing a "shrink"—they do not consider themselves "crazy" and they do not want to be labeled that way. (I take pains to assure my patients that they are not crazy but have a legitimate medical problem that is both common and treatable.)

- The waiting lists for psychiatrists, especially those who are most qualified, are often long, forcing patients to wait in their desperate condition until an appointment is available.

- Qualified and skilled psychiatrists are worth their weight in gold and accept payment accordingly. However, their hourly fee may seem outrageous to patients.

- Many psychiatrists do not accept insurance, so the patient must pay in cash at each visit.

- Primary care physicians have the best understanding of the patient's total medical history, mind and body, whereas psychiatrists, by and large, are primarily concerned with the patient's mind/brain, but may ignore the rest of the body. Full remission for most patients, however, requires the resolution of physical symptoms related to the mood disorders. This is why primary care providers are ideally positioned to make the biggest difference, such as family doctors, nurse practitioners (NPs), physician assistants (PAs), pediatricians, gynecologists, or any specialist who shows interest in recognizing and treating these mind-body disorders.

- Another example of the insurance companies' irrational perspective and priorities is that they don't cover Wellbutrin XL/Zyban (bupropion XL) if it's being given to patients to help them stop smoking because they don't cover "smoking cessation." This rule also applies to weight loss products. This is a bizarre policy that makes no sense because stopping smoking and losing weight if needed decreases health risks and thus would decrease overall health costs. This is pennywise and pound-foolish.

The obsession that causes insurance companies to fixate on the bottom-line warps their sense of reality. Their simplistic and uninformed thinking ultimately costs them more money than they save, since they could be saving more money if they had a better understanding of what goes on in a doctor's office and in the minds and bodies of their clients. If, for one minute, they were to take into consideration the fact that treating these neurochemical imbalances would result in better health and decreased risks of other medical problems, they would instantly realize the potential huge savings in overall health care. I would argue that one's insurance rates should be lower if the person is being optimally treated by the use of these preventative life-saving medications.

The problem here, however, is the persistent inability of many people throughout the entire health care community to either understand or appreciate the interrelatedness of the mind-body connection and how one can affect the other, for better or worse. By not encouraging doctors to be more involved in the treatment of conditions that are psychologically related as well as physical, insurance companies reveal their ignorance regarding the role of neurochemical imbalances as primarily *medical problems* rather than *mental problems*. If it's a mind thing then it's also necessarily a body thing too, since they cannot be separated. Doctors waste a lot of time, resources, and money sending patients off to have one test after another in search of the hidden source of their complaints, when the obvious signs of a mood disorder could more easily be diagnosed and addressed, thus cutting the cost and the time involved in patient care.

Sticking Up for Our Patients

One way doctors can get around the issue of ensuring that the patient's visit is covered rather easily is if they do not put "codes" that hint at an underlying mood disorder on a patient's "superbill" (the billing sheet that goes to the insurance companies). For example, the doctor can avoid raising suspicions with an insurance company by listing other symptoms such as headaches, insomnia, fatigue, fibromyalgia, irritable bowel syndrome, lower and upper back pain, and many other common medical symptoms that are easy to code. This is not really misleading, since most patients have at least one or two physical symptoms anyway.

The twisted nature of the managed care system—an industry that is responsible for giving people false peace of mind that they and their family will receive adequate medical attention whenever needed—is difficult to exaggerate. What can you say in defense of an institution that rewards doctors with bonuses for being "cost effective" in patient care by providing the patient with less and inferior services, procedures, and medications? I am guessing that if the general public fully knew what goes on between insurance companies and doctors who are invested in the managed-care system, there would be an outcry so loud that the government would be forced to take action.

Why are you put in the hands of a non-physician when you want to see your doctor? Because they are less expensive to hire. Why does your physician cut your visits to the shortest amount of time, not ask you questions that are pertinent to your symptoms, or not listen carefully to your complaints and the story that goes with them? Because there are no rewards for the doctors who are willing to see additional patients or spend extra time with them, listening and caring. The only incentives given doctors by the managed care companies are those that reward them for following the rules and being the most "cost effective," literally pitting doctor against patient. Hopefully, managed care will one day be a thing of the past, another one of the bad and bitter memories of our great nation.

THE MEDICAL PROFESSION: "HYPOCRITICAL OATH"?

At one time, the practice of medicine enjoyed the honor of being among the "learned professions" I mentioned earlier in this chapter. However, doctors are often disenchanted and disgruntled and have lost their passion for the profession. The end result is that patients in general suffer. A question mark hangs over the entire medical community, beginning perhaps with the American Medical

Association (AMA)—and here we discover a very ugly situation indeed.

In 1983, a secret contract between the AMA and the federal government was signed that empowered the AMA to write and publish the code book the government imposes on doctors in regard to Medicare and Medicaid billing, then other insurance companies follow suit. Doctors are required to know and abide by CPT codes (diagnosis codes), which means purchasing a new book every year and spending the time to familiarize themselves with all of its revisions from the previous year. The deal that the AMA made with the feds was that they would license the CPT to the Health Care Financing Administration (HCFA) in exchange for their agreement to not use a competing coding system, thus giving the AMA exclusive control of the codes that doctors are required to follow. Furthermore, the AMA publishes those expensive code books, which earn them more that $100,000,000 every year—more than twice the annual budget they receive through membership dues. The AMA is, therefore, responsible for the coding system that doctors must use and that is enforced by the federal government.

No wonder we find a growing cynicism and apathy among doctors regarding their profession. Since the advent of Medicare, the government has become increasingly involved in the healthcare industry, and the greatest negative impact of that involvement is felt in the examination room.

No wonder respect for this learned profession has been decreasing over the last three or four decades in proportion to the increasing regulation and paperwork demanded of doctors. A caring and skilled physician is a busy physician, but after enough intrusion by the government and insurance companies, even the most idealistic and dedicated doctor can become jaded and apathetic. They are not only distracted from their practice and time with patients, but some also may have little time (or will) left over to learn new ways of treating their patients with the greatest effectiveness. Even if they have time to learn the amazing potential of the new mood normalizing medications, they feel their hands are tied and should they attempt to be creative or innovative, they risk fines imposed by the government or a suit filed by a patient. So why take the risk? Why care? Who is taking risks for the physicians or caring for their needs and protection?

I am not, however, about to let doctors off the hook, for they have allowed corporations and the government to undermine the integrity of their profession. Now they have the responsibility to resolve these injustices. If you are tempted to think that it is impossible to battle such institutions as the AMA, insurance companies, and the federal government, then take a look at the laudable work of the Association of American Physicians and Surgeons (AAPS, http://www.aapsonline.org/). We are responsible to put up a fight and exercise more resistance to the forces that threaten the welfare of our patients.

We have already gone over the ways that physicians are told how to practice medicine, how they receive information from pharmaceutical companies regarding the use of medications, and how insurance companies seduce and bully them into reducing costs by lowering the quality of care provided to patients. For these institutions to effectively control what goes on in the doctor's office, physicians have to be compliant with all this nonsense. I am not going to minimize the pressure that is brought to bear on doctors to conform to the various standards and flawed information that is put in their faces each day, but at some point we have to take a stand for our patients. In fact, there is a lot that we can do to maneuver around the roadblocks without getting into trouble if we exercise a little creativity.

Faulty Evidence

One of the greatest weaknesses of health care today is the wide spread adoption of "Evidencebased medicine" (EBM) by physicians. In theory, EBM sounds like a good idea: Every illness and malfunction of the body and potential treatments to resolve those conditions should be subjected to the scientific method of evaluating and determining the most effective plan to follow. The problem, however, with EBM is that what gets reported in journals is often skewed by the bias of the researcher and reporter. After all, to whom will we give the authority to determine what is and is not evidence-based? I would suggest it would not be the government and insurance companies, but rather patients and doctors.

Managed care has been behind EBM, suggesting that algorithms be used to determine how doctors should treat many medical problems. I call this "cookbook medicine," which is more suited to chefs than to doctors. Then again, really good chefs do not necessarily follow the recipe line by line, but develop an *artistic feeling* for what needs to be added to the recipe, based on knowledge, experience and intuition. Guidelines, like recipes, should be treated as *suggestions* and not as mandates. Even more frightening than the interest in evidence-based medicine that managed care has shown is the federal government looking to get involved in it.

There has been an ongoing effort to restrict doctors to EBM guidelines that is in reality an effort to control (and reduce) the cost of more expensive treatments the doctor might deem necessary. If doctors were required to strictly follow guidelines laid down by researchers, even if well-intentioned, then what happens to the value of the doctor's personal experience, educated intuition, and knowledge of the individual patient? There are many variables to take into account when it comes to treating a patient, and apart from firsthand knowledge of the patient and the vital interaction with the doctor, a proper treatment plan cannot be developed. It is easy to standardize treatment protocols, but it is impossible to standardize individual patients. Doctors and not an institution, such as the government or an insurance company, are best qualified to determine what is best for the individual patient. The "art" of medicine is lost when its practice becomes regimented and overly regulated, but it is renewed when doctors are free to practice without being intimidated, harassed, or controlled.

Patients and Society: Playing the Game

We live in an ADD, quick fix, instant-gratification, and consumerist culture that has little interest in a medication that is not "fast-acting." We are to blame for our own lack of excellent health care if we have unrealistic expectations of what doctors can do, if we see them only after something has gone terribly wrong, if we look for band-aids rather than cures, and if we keep ourselves in the dark regarding what is best for us as applied to the mind and body.

Taking responsibility for our health includes the following as the bare minimum:

- The basics: nutrition, enough fluids, exercise, adequate sleep, reducing stress, and engaging in healthy and soul-enriching leisure activities.

- Insisting that our physician takes the time to hear our complaints and what we feel might be wrong with us. In many cases, the patient has proven to be right about their ailment even when, at first, the doctor cannot find any corroborating evidence.

- Insisting that our doctor explain in terms we can understand the nature of our illness and how the recommended treatment will work toward resolving it.

- Being willing to practice preventative medicine and not wait until serious problems force us to get help.

- Researching on our own the nature of our condition—whether mood disorder or other physical disorder such as diabetes—and how that condition affects and is affected by the interaction of mind and body.

- Developing a strong working relationship with our physicians regarding our health care.

- Doing what we can to support our physicians against the intrusion of institutions that have no business exerting influence over what goes on between our physicians and ourselves in the examination room or at the pharmacy.

Concluding Remarks

This chapter was a necessary addition to this book, because you need to understand why and how you have been misinformed up to the present time. If you have assumed that you could trust the FDA, AMA, your insurance carrier, or the pharmaceutical companies, I hope that you now know better. Uncovering the many cover-ups is important if we are going to move forward and make progress toward living healthier and happier lives.

The current state of our medical system is a source of deep sadness for me, and I find it very disturbing that doctors have lost control of their profession by giving too much credence and control to those who do not have the understanding of the field of medicine nor the ability to make informed and rational life-and-death decisions—not to mention their complete lack of regard for doctors and patients. The government, lawyers, managed-care organizations, and insurance companies simply do not have much in common with the cutting-edge field of medicine. In fact, the involvement of any institution with vested financial or political interests in the practice of medicine that does not result in improved quality of care necessarily results in disastrous consequences. Doctors and patients are up against some very powerful enemies that have tried to suppress the truths revealed in this book. Together we must, and will, outwit and defeat our common enemies, because our health and lives and the health of our children as well as the future for all of us depends on it.

CHAPTER EIGHT

TAKING THE "PSYCHO" OUT OF PSYCHOSOMATIC

There is a prejudice in our culture that becomes apparent when particular words are introduced to a conversation. For example, suppose two friends meet for lunch and one of them asks, "How's Joe doing?" "Oh, he's seeing a psychiatrist." What sort of assumptions do you make when you hear that statement? What if, instead of psychiatrist the friend uses another word like *psych* or *shrink?* The prejudice has to do with the outdated idea that only *crazy people* need psychiatric help.

Another word that reveals our prejudice is *psychosomatic*, which conjures images of people who create illnesses for themselves that do not really exist. We assume that a psychosomatic condition is not *real*, only *mental* and the sufferer must be mentally imbalanced and unable to cope with reality. The truth is, strictly speaking, there is not even one human experience that is not psychosomatic. So it should come as no surprise that every physical problem and symptom is connected to neurological conditions.

Psychosomatic is derived from two Greek words: *psyche*, which translates into English as *mind* or *soul* and *soma*, which is translated as *body*. Psychosomatic, therefore, refers to a state in which both the mind and body are involved, the one affecting the other.

In an earlier chapter, I explained the need to balance the complex assortment of neurochemicals in our brains to achieve optimal physical as well as mental well-being. But how does that work? That is to say, how is it that tweaking the chemistry of our brains produces harmful or beneficial effects in our bodies? The brain functions in the domain of mental states whereas the body functions in physical states, so they are two separate things, right? Actually they are not.

To keep this simple, we will avoid the muddy waters of philosophy and go straight to science. In the fields of science devoted to brain research, such as psychobiology and neuroscience, more evidence is constantly turning up that reveals the intensely complex and dynamic interplay between mental states and physical states. Everything that we see, hear, smell, touch, taste, and even think produces changes in our brain. Different neurons are activated in various parts of the brain when you perform as simple an action as looking at something.

Neurons in one part of the brain recognize patterns, shape, and size, while neurons in another part recognize color, and yet other neurons give the object a recognizable name or label.

Consider this: When you observe an orchid in bloom, leaning slightly in the wind, it is your brain that identifies the flower and can retrieve all sorts of information about flowers, including color, aroma, delicacy, and so on. But that is not all your brain does, because it is also searching its past memories and current state for an appropriate *emotional response.* If you are relatively happy, you may experience the flower with joy and a sense of gratitude. But if you have recently suffered a heartache, like the loss of someone you love, the sight of the flower may produce sadness.

The feelings we experience in response to our sensory perception of people, objects and events, reflect electrical and chemical activity in our brains. In other words, our brains are producing emotion, and at the same time our emotions affect our brain's activity. Moreover, *the neural activities in our brains are producing changes in our bodies.* In some instances, the functions of the brain produces tears, in others it may produce a smile, in danger it may produce a quick movement, in an embarrassing moment it may redden our cheeks, and so on.

Is My Condition Psychosomatic? No and Yes

Here is the important fact that we must remember: Psychosomatic conditions are *real*, having real origins and real symptoms. We are not talking about phantom pains or imaginary symptoms invented by an overly anxious mind. You see, the common misunderstanding is that physical symptoms are not real *if they are caused by mental states such as depression, stress, and anxiety*. Popular opinion is that psychosomatic illnesses involve a different set of problems than *real* medical conditions that can be identified by lab tests, probes, scans or actual visual and measurable proof that there is a problem that can be fixed. So people think, if you have an illness or injury, go see your family doctor, but if you have a psychosomatic problem, go see a psychiatrist. The truth is that the popular opinion regarding brain-induced suffering is blatantly wrong.

In communicating this information to my patients, I have to stress the fact that I take their complaints seriously. If they hear me say, "These symptoms are merely caused by stress," they will assume that I think they are *inventing* their physical problems or are just looking for attention. They also resent any hint that a professional may be implying that they are "crazy," which is how some people interpret psychosomatic conditions. So I make sure to let them know that I fully understand why they are experiencing so much suffering. The assurance and attention I give to my patients is what I am attempting to do for you, the reader, because it is possible you may have an undiagnosed (or misdiagnosed) condition. Maybe you have seen a doctor regarding an ongoing problem and have heard, "There's nothing to worry about. Take this painkiller and you'll be fine. This is a routine case of too much stress." However, if you allow your condition to be minimized, you will have to continue to bear the discomfort and perhaps despair of a problem that is likely curable.

Interconnected, Interdependent, and Entertaining

The *psyche* (mind) part of this mental-physical interaction refers to the electrical and chemical activities of the brain and the consciousness of emotions that arise as a result of those activities. The *soma* (body) part of the interaction is the body's role in perceiving external and internal sensations, relaying them to the brain and then responding to whatever commands the brain issues in order to make adjustments to those sensations. Of course, the brain has to interpret the signals from the body based on past experience and other resident or stored information, and it has only milliseconds in which to do it.

If the brain and each of its delicate systems are not operating as they should, a malfunction or multiple malfunctions will occur. In regard to the *psyche*, patients will experience the malfunction emotionally in terms of depression, anxiety, agitation, and so on. In regard to the *soma*, patients are likely to suffer symptoms, such as nausea, stomachaches, headaches, and so on. You already know where your body carries the strain and stress of your brain. For example, if you find yourself rubbing the back of your neck at the end of a stressful day, rolling your shoulders to ease the muscle tension, taking something to relieve a headache or settle your stomach, or checking your heart rate or blood pressure, then you have located the point (or points) where your body responds to what your brain is trying to address.

How is it that mental and emotional factors can register in the body as *physical* symptoms? The answer is the complete unity of the brain, nervous system, and body, which function as one whole organism. What is more, is the realization we need to face that, because of the increased pace of life, growing number of daily decisions we must make, and intensification of personal and world problems, a greater number of people are struck by these conditions every year–*normal people!* To the intensity of life's demands we must also add the breakdown of traditional support systems, such as faith, family, and community.

The Most Common (and Treatable) Psychosomatic Conditions

The remainder of the chapter will highlight conditions we hear about every day that are related to the mind-body connection. In some cases, the problem begins with emotional and stress issues, while in other cases it begins in the body, but in either case, the interplay between mind and body means that both will be affected and each will influence the other. The point that I want to underscore in this section is that the most unrecognized, and therefore undiagnosed and untreated malfunctions in these conditions are the chemical imbalances in the brain that are *caused by* or are the *cause of* the emotional and physical symptoms.

Chronic Fatigue Syndrome (CFS)

Many of my patients who suffer from Chronic Fatigue Syndrome (CFS) have seen other doctors and specialists before they arrive at my office. They come to me frustrated and complaining that, "No one has figured out why I am so tired all of the time." They have exhausted (no pun intended) all leads, some have read all the reports on the Internet, and may have attempted multiple cures without getting any better. Some of them have attempted to heal themselves with *natural* supplements. Unfortunately, they have only minimal results. Others have attempted to apply band-aids to their symptoms that fail over time or even create a worse situation.

In the case of some CFS patients, the presence of a mood disorder is immediately obvious, while other patients' indications are more subtle. The typical attempts to diagnose CFS that have endured include panels that test for Epstein-Barr virus and other viral tests, blood counts to rule out iron or vitamin B12 deficiency, thyroid function, endocrine issues such as hormonal levels, and other results that are often unnecessary and usually unrevealing anyway. This is assuming, of course, that doctors have ruled out organ failures or other diseases that could account for loss of energy. Even if a previous doctor believes he or she has discovered "medical confirmation" of CFS, the treatments may not have produced the result they wanted most: Increased energy.

The reason why blood panels and other tests are not always successful in diagnosing and addressing CFS is because in many instances this condition is related to a chemical imbalance. At present, there are no accurate clinical tests that reveal the status of neurochemicals in the brain. The most practical and effective way to test for chemical imbalances is to give patients samples of medications that are most likely to address CFS. If it works, then I was right. If it doesn't work, then I was wrong. The medication trial is, therefore, both the diagnostic test and the treatment at the same time. This is unique in the medical field. Of course, I will prescribe a blood panel if a work up has not yet been done or the medications do not produce the changes I anticipate within a reasonable period of time.

Medications that balance a person's neurochemicals provide a feeling of natural energy and not the fake boost that comes through amphetamines or the wide variety of caffeine-laden "energy drinks." The real and natural energy that follows the balancing of neurochemicals through safe and effective medications makes people feel like "their old selves" again or even better.

Mood-normalizing medications are usually a necessary part of the treatment, but never the whole treatment. For all humans, a decent diet and regular exercise are necessary to maintain optimum levels of energy. People who are energy-deficient would be wise also to monitor their intake of simple carbohydrates and sugars.

Neurochemicals to address in the following order:

- Dopamine
- Norepinephrine
- GABA
- Serotonin

In some cases, the condition will be resolved once dopamine has been properly balanced requiring Wellbutrin XL (bupropion XL) by itself in rare cases. If dopamine is an issue, then norepinephrine as well as the other neurochemicals may also need to be balanced in order to provide the best results.

An SNRI could be useful in this situation, usually in augmentation, since the right cocktail of medications tends to provide the most complete results. Adding Nuvigil (armodafinil)/Provigil (modafinil), Deplin (L-methylfolate) and/or a stimulant can also be considered, if needed and if it is tolerated.

As always, every individual is different, so there will be a certain amount of diagnosis and treatment through trial and error. Nevertheless, the indications of the disorder and the medications chosen to address it can and should be approached rationally.

There is no greater reward than to witness the excitement and joy of patients as their energy level is restored and, in turn, their lives are changed. This is especially true in cases where the patient has suffered with CFS for some time. Armed with this knowledge that together we have found a treatment program that is *natural* and *preventative* gives me the satisfaction of not only knowing they are *feeling* better, but that they are *becoming* better, healthier, and more whole because we have confronted the real problem and not merely laid a band-aid over it.

FIBROMYALGIA

Like those patients who suffer from Chronic Fatigue, most Fibromyalgia patients have traveled a long and frustrating journey from doctor, to lab, to nutritionist, and anyone else who offers them hope of relief. The primary reason for the run around is due to the difficulty doctors have in diagnosing this condition. Fibromyalgia is sort of a *last resort* diagnosis after conditions that cause some of the same symptoms have been ruled out. Besides symptoms like sleep disorders and irritable bowel syndrome, the most sinister symptom is the widespread pain a patient experiences in muscles, joints, and soft tissue. There may be some places on the patient's body that are tender and painful to the touch, but those are only the most acute locations. The pain sometimes feels like it is coming from everywhere at once.

There are potential hidden and life-threatening problems that can be masked by the pain that should be looked into if needed, though much of the testing that a Fibromyalgia patient has had to endure is mostly unnecessary. Even while running the other tests, a doctor who suspects early on that Fibromyalgia may be the culprit can begin applying mood-normalizing medications to the problem as a means of diagnosis and treatment at the same time. In other words, if the patient shows a quick and positive response to a medication or combinations of medications, then the doctor has taken a major step forward in the diagnosis.

I have seen doctors and nurses roll their eyes when a patient announces that she has Fibromyalgia. This is because it is common medical knowledge that stress plays a central role in the flare-up of symptoms. Some professionals assume that they are dealing with highly emotional, uptight, or overly anxious patients who are probably making their condition worse by constantly obsessing over it. Others consider the condition to be purely psychological and refer patients with fibromyalgia to psychologists.

Patients can usually discern when their physician has adopted a condescending attitude toward them. If a doctor, office staff or other healthcare workers become judgmental towards a patient, they have not only clouded their reason, but they forfeit the opportunity to be agents of healing. As we have seen, psychosomatic illnesses are neither purely this or purely that, but are mental and physical at the same time. Fibromyalgia is a real condition, the pain is real, and the best approach to treatment is to help the patient begin to hope through sincere concern, listening, and affirmation.

The experience of pain in our bodies is perceived by local neurons that relay information to the brain. Chemical imbalances affect the nerves that supply muscles, ligaments, tendons, joints, skin, and other tissues and can cause inflammation that results in pain, but can also trigger other symptoms such as muscle contraction or spasms that intensify the pain. If the doctor and patient are able to work together to balance the right neurochemicals, they can eliminate the inflammation and potentially reduce or completely resolve the pain.

Unfortunately, in many cases there are a lot of narcotics, muscle relaxants, anti-inflammatory medications, and other pain medications applied to fibromyalgia. The problem though is that some of these medications are potentially addictive and most of them are rarely necessary, except for the more acute pain. I have seen many patients discontinue the band-aid application of drugs to symptoms when the burden of fibromyalgia was relieved by addressing the source of the problem. Sometimes people are under the spell of our *quick fix* culture and want the immediate relief of symptoms even though in the long term they are doing more damage to themselves than good. We want to think we can be healthy without moderate exercise—and in the case of fibromyalgia, a good program of stretching and cardiovascular exercise is very helpful. Having a balanced diet also helps. Our bodies were made to be treated with a certain amount of respect for the way they naturally develop, mend, and heal. To ignore the body's basic immune system, and what keeps it in good working order, is to guarantee serious problems down the road. Mood normalizing medications frequently play a key role in assisting the natural processes of the body's healing mechanisms.

Neurochemicals to address in the following order:

- Norepinephrine
- GABA
- Dopamine
- Serotonin

Combining medications is the rule, since in the majority of cases in which there is recurring pain, more than one neurochemical is imbalanced.

An SNRI-GABAergic medication such as Topamax (topiramate) or Neurontin (gabapentin) is a common combination I put together for somatic/pain symptoms. Regardless of which strategy works best, once the chemicals are in balance, the patient's quality of life is dramatically improved, because living with unnecessary pain is not really living.

HEADACHES

The most common cause of acute and chronic headaches, whether muscular, migraine, or a combination, is *stress*. Muscular or tension headaches are the most common by far. A chemical imbalance affecting the nerve supply in the scalp, neck, and upper back muscles can result in everything from mild to severe headaches. I often show patients where their neck muscles attach to the "bumps" at the lower back of the skull where the bones, ligaments, and muscles come together, which is a common area of pain. These muscles thin out and wrap around the skull, making their way to the forehead and the entire face. If something causes these muscles to contract more than what is normal or necessary, they can create a squeezing sensation that, to headache patients, feels like their head is in a vise grip and is being slowly squeezed.

Migraine headaches are also commonly caused by an imbalance of chemicals within nerves that are attached to blood vessels, causing abnormal constriction and dilation. This is what creates the *pulsating and throbbing sensation* of migraine headaches. The migraine can occur on either side of the head or both sides at the same time. The "classic" migraines, with or without an aura, are often one-sided. Nausea is also a classic symptom with migraine headaches, which is not typically the case with tension/muscular headaches.

Although the most common cause of migraines is physical or emotional stress, other things, such as the ingestion of certain foods, atmospheric and barometric changes, humidity changes, allergies, hormonal changes, and other environmental factors, can also bring them on.

Neurochemicals to address in the following order:

- Norepinephrine (as in the case of fibromyalgia and other pain syndromes).
- GABA
- Dopamine
- Serotonin

As always, prevention is my number one concern. Besides preventative medications such as SNRIs over SSRIs and GABAergic medications such as Topamax or Gabapentin, I cannot overemphasize the miraculous benefits of regular exercise with stretching and relaxation techniques.

Sadly, many people struggle through life battling ongoing, debilitating headaches. Frustrated by fruitless attempts to resolve this problem, some have thrown in the towel, saying, "I guess that's just the way my life is going to be." Perhaps that is the way the lives of some people will go, but I assure you, that is not the way life is *supposed* to be.

Chronic Pain Syndromes

Chemical imbalances are responsible for many of the general conditions of ongoing pain in the head, neck, upper and lower back muscles, chest muscles, abdominal muscles, muscles of the arms and legs, around the lining of the lungs (sharp pleurisy-like chest pain), around the sternum (breast bone) referred to as costochondritis, and a variety of other areas around the body. The reason mood normalizing medications work so well for resolving pain is because nerves go everywhere *throughout* the body (every cell in the body has a nerve close to it). Balancing and calming the nerves serves as a chain reaction, since the nerves then calm the tissues to which they are attached.

Even when X-rays or other tests reveal a structural cause for pain, we cannot rule out the fact that stress still plays a role and, in fact, is the primary reason why pain flares up when it does. Massaging, even injecting, areas where structural issues are present will usually help for the short-term only. However, getting the neurochemicals in proper balance is a better approach for long-term healing.

You may be interested in learning that many patients with autoimmune diseases, such as lupus, rheumatoid arthritis, Sjögren's syndrome, and so on, have experienced significant improvement through the use of mood normalizing medications by the prevention of inflammation caused by these conditions. Some patients have dramatically reduced the use of anti-inflammatories and pain pills when taking mood normalizing medications, which gives the healing process a significant boost, thus improving the outcome of other treatments that address autoimmune disease.

I'll never forget the woman I saw with severe crippling RA (rheumatoid arthritis) who had joint disfigurement and a lot of pain. Within weeks after an SNRI-GABA combo her pain was at least 80-90% better. Her rheumatologist was able to drastically decrease her pain pills (opiates and anti-inflammatories) and stop the corticosteroid prednisone. He called me to inquire how I did that and why the psychotropics were making such a dramatic difference. After I explained it to him he said, "Wow. I probably should do that with most of my patients!"

Patients with chronic pain may get the greatest benefit if they adopt a *team approach* to their pain by working with physical therapists, psychologists, acupuncturists, and pain specialists, if needed. Otherwise, the medication options for treating chronic pain syndromes are the same as those for treating headaches and fibromyalgia. No matter what it takes, doctors and patients should use whatever is available and whatever is required to subdue and prevent pain, because pain itself is a cause of stress, and stress exacerbates pain. Seeing that we have the ability to break this vicious cycle, why not?

Skin Symptoms

By now you can probably figure out on your own that the skin that wraps our bodies is serviced by the nervous system. Therefore, chemical imbalances related to mood disorders can cause reactions in the skin, some chronic (such as eczema), some annoying (like itchy rashes), some that are dangerous, and some that are extremely painful. Many people are very much aware of the fact that when they have been under a great deal of stress or have been plagued with anxiety, their skin responds by breaking out with hives or acne.

The skin is the largest organ and our bodies' first line of defense, and everyday it is bombarded by bacteria, viruses, fungi, and others that are constantly present in our environment. Herpes simplex and Herpes Zoster (shingles) are common skin infections, which can be painful. Normally, when we are healthy and at peace, our immune system can ward off the vast majority of infectious attacks. Ongoing stress, depression and anxiety, however, can wear down the immune system and leave the skin more vulnerable to whatever microbes happen to land on it. When the immune system isn't functioning properly, the patient is not only subjected to greater suffering, but runs the risk of their condition becoming systemic. The best treatment is prevention by maintaining the balance of neurons that supply the skin.

Sexual Dysfunction

Sexual function is directly related to optimal mental and physical health. Stress leading to a neurochemical imbalance or vice versa should be considered as a significant culprit in such problems as low libido, delayed orgasm, anorgasmia, the inability to achieve orgasm (no payoff at the end), erectile dysfunction, and premature ejaculation. Of course, there are other organic causes that can contribute to these problems, and those other diagnosed conditions should first be considered and addressed if needed. Psychological reasons for sexual problems are more common than physical causes, though for some it may be a combination of both.

Some of the medications that are available to treat premature ejaculation (most commonly an SSRI) can, at the same time, potentially cause sexual problems for men or women. Though mood normalizing agents may cause these side effects, this is usually resolvable. For many they actually improve functioning because people who feel better about themselves enjoy sex more.

Dopamine is the first chemical to consider as being imbalanced, with Wellbutrin (bupropion) being the treatment of choice, though the others may also be involved. Medications are not the only option in the case of sexual dysfunction. Weight control is a very important issue. Being overweight can lower male (and female) libido, especially in men and women over forty to fifty years of age, though younger people can also be affected. It is important to have a well-balanced diet, participate in regular exercise, quit smoking, moderation of alcohol use, treatment of diabetes, hypertension and high cholesterol, thyroid imbalance, low testosterone, and proper attention to other medical needs. Open communication between partners is very important, and counseling may be helpful if needed. Any of these treatments can be effective independently of the others and all of them can be effective working harmoniously together, and they have one common goal: To reduce stress on the mind and body as much as possible to achieve optimal sexual functioning for each individual.

HORMONAL SYMPTOMS

I frequently hear parents talk about their hormonally charged-up teenagers, and how they so easily spin out of control—lots of drama one day, sullen and withdrawn the next, sleeping through the following day, and so on. What is less well understood, and yet critically important, is that adolescence is not the only stage in our lives when we experience hormonal changes. Not only do we undergo age-related changes at various stages of life (e.g., menopause), but fluctuations in hormone levels can also be caused by natural and traumatic events (e.g., pregnancy, injury or illness).

Every alteration in our hormonal balance creates the potential for an alteration to the chemistry of our nervous system. The blade can also swing in the other direction when neurochemical changes trigger hormonal changes. As a result, people with no previous history of a mood disorder, such as depression, can become sullen and hopeless almost overnight. The reverse can also occur, when a person who has struggled for years with depression suddenly becomes hopeful and positive. This particular change is referred to as *spontaneous remission.*

PREMENSTRUAL SYNDROME (PMS)

Hormonal fluctuations can be frustrating because they arrive so abruptly. Neither the person nor those close to them understand how one day everything can seem perfectly fine and harmonious and the next day the individual has had a sudden mood swing, is inexplicably irritable and impatient, listless and apathetic. Although we sometimes hear comedians and others joke about PMS, there is nothing funny to the women who suffer from premenstrual syndrome or more properly called premenstrual dysphoric disorder (PMDD). When estrogen levels dip after ovulation and prior to the onset of menses, simultaneous imbalances of serotonin and other neurochemicals frequently follow. Shifting emotions and physical symptoms, such as headaches and stomach cramps, can begin up to two weeks before a woman's period, more commonly within a few days to a week or so prior. Similar symptoms also occur during other peak times of hormonal changes.

Naturally, doctors are concerned about the fluctuation of hormones during these times of changes, but to treat the whole person they need to consider addressing the possibility of a neurochemical imbalance as well. For example, a woman may receive a prescription for "The Pill" or Hormone Replacement Therapy (HRT), which may correct the hormonal component of her condition, yet likely will fail to resolve the neurochemical component.

Mood normalizing medications have proven to be very helpful during the difficult times of hormonal changes. In fact, one option available to doctors and patients is to use the medication only during the days of hormonal changes, since they work almost immediately on these days. Some women have discovered that when they are on medication for two weeks prior to menstruation, they actually feel better on their PMS days than they do the rest of the month. I may then just try continuing the medication the rest of the month to see how she responds. What this response indicates is a basic chemical imbalance that had not been recognized, but needed to be addressed all along.

Another option is to take the medications all month if the mood changes are not limited to a specific period of time prior to menstruations. The dosage of medication can also be adjusted up for the critical days when they are most needed (the Luteal phase), but backed down again the rest of the month (the follicular phase). Going a step further, different medications can be used on different days depending on a woman's response to each medication and her particular needs. As we have seen again and again, each person is unique and the doctor and patient have to work together to determine the specific treatment that the individual's condition requires.

Irritable Bowel Syndrome (IBS)

The source of many problems that patients suffer from, such as pain or recurring abnormalities within the stomach, intestinal and digestive tracts, can be traced back to a chemical imbalance in many. It may be necessary to rule out any apparent cause, such as those that would show up in an external examination, x-ray, or endoscope (an instrument that allows doctors to look at the inside of the intestines or exterior of the organs inside the body). However, when colonoscopies, scans, stool studies, blood workups and other lab tests do not yield a substantial diagnosis, we can be fairly certain that a chemical imbalance is at the root of the problem. Irritable Bowel Syndrome is another "rule out" diagnosis (like Fibromyalgia), in so much as it is the name doctors will give to a condition that cannot otherwise be diagnosed and may include the following: bloating, gas, cramping, diarrhea, constipation, and pain.

I need to also add this important word of advice to doctors and patients: There is no need to wait for a complete diagnostic work up before beginning treatment with mood normalizing medications. Even if a serious organic cause of the symptoms is discovered, the medications will not have done the patient any harm and are likely to do them good in relieving some of their anxiety regarding the outcome of the diagnostic tests. In fact, most patients find the time period between undergoing the tests and learning the results to be more excruciating than their symptoms. If the medications resolve the symptoms, then they have proven to be a useful diagnostic tool indeed. These are not "pain medications," so they will not *mask* a physical condition. Rather, they may likely prevent the pain from happening in the first place.

Nerves supply the muscles and tissues that surround each loop of the intestines as well as the muscles and glands of the stomach. If the chemicals in these nerves are imbalanced, the functions of the lower GI tract will be affected, which can result in abnormal constriction and dilation of the intestines. This should create a smooth, coordinated and rhythmic movement of the intestines (called peristalsis) in the elimination of waste. If the orderly massaging effect of the intestinal muscles is disrupted by nerves that are not properly served, due to a chemical imbalance, a number of other problems can develop along with a variety of symptoms that can make the patient's life miserable, such as spasms, inflammation and pain.

Inflammatory Bowel Disease (IBD) such as Crohn's disease and ulcerative colitis are often responsive to the preventative approach that applies mood-normalizing medications to chemical imbalances. One of the rationales behind this form of treatment has to do with the fact that stress can be not only the cause of the problem, but can also trigger and intensify flare-ups of these conditions. Most patients also respond to the flare-ups with more stress, knowing that they are going to have to ride out the pain and put up with the treatment, and this can make it last longer and occur more frequently. Addressing the chemical imbalance not only decreases and diminishes the flare-ups, it also seems to improve the immune system by decreasing the demand that is made on it by a malfunctioning and stress-inducing digestive system.

As always, there is no escaping the fact that if you want to enjoy optimum physical and mental health, a well-balanced diet and regular exercise are not negotiable. In regard to IBS, this regimen would also include adequate fiber intake and aerobic exercises to improve metabolism and abdominal musculature (e.g., "core" training).

Doctors who prescribe medications such as Librium (chlordiazepoxide hydrochloride) and Valium (diazepam) and other "bowel tranquilizers" for IBS are merely applying band-aids. Those who treat IBS with laxatives, multiple fiber supplements, suppositories, enemas, and "bowel cleansings" usually achieve no more than temporary relief.

Neurochemicals to address in the following order:

- Norepinephrine
- Serotonin
- GABA
- Dopamine

If you or someone you know has suffered from IBS, take heart. Relief and prevention are not only achievable, but are likely to occur with medications that are readily available.

INSOMNIA

The term *insomnia* is used to describe a number of sleeping disorders that include difficulty in falling asleep (delayed sleep-phase syndrome), interruption of sleep with difficulty falling back to sleep, waking up too early, and so on. One of the primary indicators of insomnia is that the sleep time allotted does not leave the person refreshed. In all but the rarest cases, chronic recurring insomnia can be resolved by balancing neurochemicals.

Mood disorders, such as depression and anxiety, are known to have a direct effect on sleep patterns, either causing a person to sleep too much or too little. In turn, insomnia tends to worsen or aggravate mood disorders. In the case of bipolar disorder, sleep is interrupted by restlessness due to the mind's frenetic racing or by the patient's feeling that sleep is unnecessary.

Beside the use of medications, there are some basic conditions that can be created around sleep time to optimize its effectiveness in muscle and tissue recovery as well as our overall rest. I refer to this as good sleep hygiene.

These conditions would include:

1. Making certain that the bedroom is as dark and quiet as possible.

2. Do not allow your bed to become a couch, desk, snack area, or reading table, but reserve it for sleep and sex. In this way we condition our minds to expect to fall asleep when we crawl into bed.

3. Get at least a half hour of vigorous exercise during the day.

4. Learn simple relaxation techniques to help induce sleep at bedtime.

5. Avoid mental and physical stimulation from such activities as suspenseful books, television shows, or movies, or exercise too close to bedtime.

6. Avoid self-medicating ways of "knocking yourself out" at night. Alcohol, for example, is a well-known source of sleep disturbances. Insomnia is commonly addressed by patients and doctors with band-aid treatments, such as prescription sleeping pills, tranquilizers, muscle relaxants, alcohol, street drugs or by "prescription," and over-the-counter sleeping aids, but I have found that mood-normalizing medications are the best way to reset the clock (the brain's normal rhythms) and restore a normal sleep pattern. If you feel that you *need* "band aid" prescription medications, "herbal remedies," or alcohol in order to fall asleep, you have a sure sign that a chemical imbalance is at the root of your insomnia.

Our goal in treating insomnia is to recover a normal sleeping pattern through a proper balance of neurochemicals that are necessary for good rest. In particular, we are interested in improving the quality of REM sleep, because this is crucial to refreshing both the mind and body.

Neurochemicals to address in the following order:

- Norepinephrine
- Dopamine
- GABA
- Serotonin

The reality for most is that a combination of agents is likely to work best because insomnia results from an imbalance of more than one neurochemical.

HYPERTENSION

Most people are aware of the way stress can raise their blood pressure. In fact, I have seen patients whose blood pressure rises significantly when their blood pressure is taken simply because they are worried about what the test will say. "White coat" phenomenon results in elevated blood pressure due to the patient's nervousness. When diagnosing high blood pressure, a doctor must first determine the role played by "primary" hypertension and then the role played by secondary causes. So the doctor and patient will compile a patient-history based on family background, a review of charted blood pressure results that patients keep while monitoring their blood pressure at home, a basic lab workup, looking for other medical conditions that may contribute to it, an EKG, and obtaining a cardiology consultation for a stress test if needed.

Mood normalizing medications can produce dramatic improvements in patients with high blood pressure, and especially in cases where the condition is either caused or intensified by emotional stress. Some of my patients have been able to reduce or even discontinue use of blood pressure medications after resolving the chemical imbalance that contributes to their stress and high blood pressure.

Mood normalizing medications "kill two birds with one stone" when they assist the mind and the body at the same time. The medications should be started at a low dosage while closely monitoring the patient's progress and gradually increasing the doses until the desired results are achieved.

The conventional blood pressure medications are still very important and are useful in keeping the heart and body functioning optimally in individuals with high blood pressure. However, because mood disorders and chemical imbalances are found alongside other medical conditions more often than not, mood normalizing medications may increase the effectiveness of other treatment options or prevent other medications from being needed in the first place. I have had several patients stop blood pressure medications without negative consequences, though this requires close monitoring. This is simply good medicine, when doctors and patients work closely to address the issues of both mind and body, since the one necessarily affects the other.

Neurological and Circulatory Changes

Neurological and circulatory changes include numbness and tingling (paresthesias), muscle inflammation and spasms, tremors, pain, and decreased circulation of the smallest distal blood vessels affecting fingers/hands and toes/feet, etc. ("Raynaud's" phenomenon). Because these symptoms are difficult to classify and explain, we should immediately suspect that a neurochemical imbalance is the culprit. Chemical imbalances of the nerves that are attached to the muscles and tissues throughout the body can cause them to become irritated and create these unpleasant symptoms.

Restless leg syndrome (RLS) is an extremely unpleasant condition for people who suffer from it. It is manifested by frequent leg movements that happen involuntarily, especially when trying to wind down and go to sleep. It can also result in disruption of sleep, and other conditions that result in muscular spasm, inflammation, and pain, which can also result from a chemical imbalance of the nerves supplying these muscles. These symptoms tend to increase at night and during more restful times of the day since anxiety and stress stored in the body tend to manifest during these times, when the body internally is not ready to rest.

Circulatory changes are also affected by mood. Anxiety increases epinephrine (adrenaline) within the nervous system, which can change the flow of blood within the blood vessels. This particular chemical imbalance causes blood vessels to constrict and dilate, which in turn decreases and increases the flow of blood to the tissue it is servicing.

Diagnosis of neurological and circulatory conditions begin with a physical exam, a blood panel, and a basic workup to rule out the more obvious medical causes for the symptoms. Some patients will be referred to a neurologist or cardiologist for consultation and further testing. If no obvious cause shows up to make a diagnosis or current symptoms are unexplained and unresolved, a trial using mood normalizing medications is the best step to take next in the diagnostic and treatment process.

Tranquilizers, muscle relaxants, medications that slow down the heart rate, and other medications that are intended only to relieve symptoms may cause fatigue, which could worsen mood and produce other side effects. Besides, if mood-normalizing medications are effective, these others will not be needed.

Exercise and relaxation techniques, including prayer and meditation, are great stress reducers, and improve the cardiovascular, nervous, and immune systems that help the mind and the body achieve a state of rest. A person who is more active will be less likely to succumb to stress than a person who does not get regular exercise.

Dizziness

Although we tend to take it for granted, keeping our body balanced is an extremely complex process that depends on some of the smallest and most delicate instruments ever discovered. If you have ever stood up too fast after being at rest in a prone position and seen stars, become dizzy, or nearly fainted, then you are aware of how quickly and easily the mechanisms on which your brain relies can be disabled.

To oversimplify the balancing mechanism of the inner ear, imagine a laboratory where there are several plastic tubes suspended on a hinge so that they can rock up and down like a teeter-totter. Each tube is filled with a thick fluid and inside the tubes there are small flexible filaments so that if a tube is tipped up on one side and the fluid flows downward to the other side, the filament is moved by the liquid. Every time the filament moves, it relays a signal to a computer that records and interprets the motion. At all times the computer tracks the movements of the fluid and makes necessary adjustments based on that information.

That, basically, is how the brain is able to orient itself and the body is able to maintain balance. Any motion of the body, or even merely tipping the head, causes fluid inside small cavities in the skull to flow around. When the tiny hairs in those cavities are moved by the fluid, the nerve impulses they send to the brain are either increased or decreased.

The brain reads and interprets these messages and responds accordingly. The balancing process can be affected by something as simple as rapidly twirling in circles, as most children very well know.

The nerves that communicate from the inner ear where the mechanisms of balance are located can be affected by a chemical imbalance. Dizziness, vertigo, hypersensitivity that results in visual changes, tinnitus (ringing of the ears), and other balanced-related conditions are all symptomatic of problems that affect those nerves. The inner ear is susceptible to impairment from injury, illness, and any changes in the circulatory or nervous systems.

Hyperventilation and other changes in the breathing pattern can also affect balancing mechanisms. Some people breathe too rapidly when they are nervous, frightened, or worried, and most of these people do not even realize that their breathing pattern has changed. Not only do they breathe too fast, but they tend to take shallow breaths, which prevents the carbon dioxide from exhaling before the next breath of oxygen is inhaled. The results of erratic breathing include oxygen deprivation and changes in circulation and the nervous system, which can produce dizziness and the other symptoms mentioned.

Relaxation techniques and slow deep breathing (i.e.: "paper bag" breathing) are the typical strategies for immediately responding to hyperventilation. Cardiovascular exercise is very helpful in treating hyperventilation, but it is important to make certain that the person is safe and not at risk of fainting and falling.

Addressing only the symptoms of balance-related problems, doctors usually rely on Antivert/meclizine and minor tranquilizers such as Valium or others. I have found that a better approach is to address the real underlying problem instead.

Hair Loss

To date there is no effective way to prevent or reverse the normal process of male-pattern baldness. The three conditions that determine whether a man will experience hair loss are heredity (twenty-three chromosomes from the father and twenty-three from the mother), male hormone, and age.

Anyone though, male or female, can experience an abnormal thinning of the hair that can result from illness or aggressive treatment of disease. Abnormal hair loss can also occur during times of intense stress, when a person's hair begins falling out at a faster rate than it is replaced. Other less common reasons for abnormal hair loss are thyroid imbalance, nutritional deficiencies, and primary skin disorders. However, anxiety and stress are the most common causes of unusual thinning.

I have observed that stress-related hair loss can begin two to three months after the peak of acute stress and last for however long the patient remains in a stress-inducing situation. About the same period of time, two to three months, after the stress has resolved, or if the patient has received help in developing ways to cope with stress, hair will start to fill back in and return to its normal cycles. These are rough estimates since the precise amount of time required for new hair growth depends on the specifics of each individual case. When a patient's hair growth returns to normal, the doctor and patient have visible evidence that the mental and physical stress has been relieved. Because many people panic when they notice that their hair is thinning, they are greatly comforted to learn that it is frequently a temporary condition and can be addressed by mood-normalizing medications if needed.

URINARY SYMPTOMS

Chemical changes within the nerves supplying the bladder can cause hyperactivity and hypersensitivity of the nerves. This may result in either a "nervous bladder" with increased urinary frequency or inflammation and pain of the bladder caused by interstitial cystitis and other disorders. There is a class of medications called tricyclic antidepressants (Elavil, Pamelor, or others in this class) which have been used for years for bladder incontinence and symptoms of bladder irritability, frequency, and inflammation. The reason they can be so effective is that they balance both serotonin and norepinephrine at the same time, which is why I refer to them as the "primitive" SNRI's (medications that inhibit the abnormal reuptake of serotonin and norepinephrine). Adding a low-dose tricyclic to an SSRI has been a strategy used for many years by pain specialists and primary-care doctors. The four more modern SNRIs are the best first-line treatment choices that work better and are better tolerated. I have also found that balancing one's neurochemicals may also help to balance estrogen and other hormones which may result in the strengthening of the muscles and other tissues surrounding the bladder and its outflow.

One symptom of anxiety is dry mouth, which can result in increased thirst with resultant increased fluid intake. This in turn may contribute to increased urinary frequency with resultant increased symptoms of bladder spasms, inflammation, and pain.

Urinary, gastrointestinal symptoms and headaches are common complaints with children when they are under stress. Headaches and gastrointestinal problems especially are the most common causes for missed school, if school is one of the sources of stress that brings out these symptoms. I have noted that some adults who, as a child, had problems with stool retention, constipation, and bowel irregularities, may be more likely to turn into "anal-retentive" adults (those that are very uptight). They seem to internalize stress more, which causes them to be more sensitive to this as well as other stress-related symptoms in general due to underlying neurochemical imbalances that are in need of being corrected.

GASTROINTESTINAL REFLUX
(ACID REFLUX/PEPTIC ULCER DISEASE)

Gastrointestinal symptoms are a common problem that can manifest when anxiety is the underlying cause. Stress can increase the production of acid in the stomach, which can lead to reflux into the esophagus and erosion of the stomach lining. Even if peptic ulcer disease were caused by the bacterial infection *Helicobacter pylori*, it would make sense that treating the underlying neurochemical imbalances, if needed, would improve the immune system so the infection would be more easily contained. Moreover, the production of acid would decrease, thereby improving the function of the stomach in general.

A "nervous stomach" can be present due to increased acid production internally and irritation from the stomach externally due to an imbalance of the nerves supplying it with resultant inflammation and spasm of the muscles surrounding it. This may be the result of imbalances chemically within the nerves supplying these areas, which can be corrected. These symptoms are often medicated by antacids and H2 (histamine 2) blockers (Zantac, Pepcid, Axid, Tagamet, and PPIs (proton pump inhibitors) such as Prilosec, Nexium, Aciphex, Prevacid and Protonix. They are also medicated through stomach and intestinal symptomatic medications, such as tranquilizers, pain pills, gas-reducing agents, as well as other symptomatic medications, such as Levin/levbid, bentyl or others, which can help to decrease bloating and pain. A preventative approach toward correcting the underlying anxiety can result in normalization of acid production and bowel motility with mood-normalizing medications with resultant improvement of stomach symptoms. I have often seen people able to stop all symptomatic medications once prevention is optimized. This preventative and more holistic approach can also be more cost effective, since less use of symptomatic medications can save money in the long run. Decreasing stress in general provides for a better gastrointestinal environment, both upper and lower, thus leading to an improved quality of life.

Chronic Recurring Infections

Stress not only makes one more prone to infections but also causes those infections to last longer and to be more resistant to treatment by interfering with a healthy immune system. Well-known examples include "cold sores" (caused by herpes simplex and other viruses) and shingles (herpes zoster virus). I have also seen this phenomenon at play with other types of infections, such as bronchitis, sinusitis, urinary tract infections, skin infections, as well as other infections.

When people are under stress they are more likely to succumb when exposed to viruses, bacteria, fungi, parasites, or other types of infections, which eventually can result in inflammation and infection of whichever part of the body the nerves are supplying. Proper balancing of one's neurochemicals, if needed, is the best preventative way to improve not only the immune system, but also one's overall health.

Bruxism (Teeth Grinding)

The grinding of one's teeth is a common symptom that is often related to unresolved stress. Those who don't adequately relieve stress during the daytime are more likely to tense their jaws and grind their teeth at night. This is because the body is trying to relax but is not able to because of underlying muscular tension, which can transfer to the jaw, gums and teeth. This is because the mind is still going, and this causes restless sleep and bad dreams with resultant tension of the mouth and jaw. This can lead to TMJ strain with recurrent jaw pain and headaches. My dentist told me that some of his patients have actually fractured their teeth because of bruxism, and that this can cause other damage to the teeth requiring more dental procedures and interventions. Addressing the underlying stress can improve and resolve this symptom, which can also reduce stress by reducing the number of visits to the dentist and the associated costs and discomfort.

Respiratory Symptoms

Stress not only affects the circulatory system, but also the respiratory system, since nerves also innervate the lungs. A chemical imbalance within these nerves can create symptoms, such as hyperventilation and shortness of breath. When the respiratory rate and depth of respirations are affected, this can create an imbalance of oxygen and carbon dioxide which, in turn, can lead to other symptoms, such as dizziness, paresthesias (numbness and tingling), and palpitations. I have also seen that increased stress brings increased and worsened episodes of asthma. These asthma symptoms can then increase anxiety, which then creates more symptoms, and so on. Balancing the chemicals within the nerves can resolve the anxiety thereby breaking this vicious cycle by normalizing breathing and helping patients feel normal.

Palpitations

Irregular heart rate, or the perception of this, and tachycardia (increased heart rate) are common symptoms potentially related to anxiety. These symptoms can hit close to home, and can fuel fears of having actual heart disease as the adrenaline surges abnormally due to the underlying imbalance within the nervous system. This may then stimulate the heart's electrical system, causing irregularities in the heart rate. Blood pressure can also increase and decrease quickly due to abnormal constriction and dilation of the blood vessels from the heart as well as those supplying the heart muscle and the heart's nervous system.

These symptoms lead to increased anxiety, which results in more symptoms, and this may cause one to speculate about the symptoms of a heart attack and wonder if that is what is going on now. They recall it has to do with chest pain, which they are experiencing, and has something to do with left arm symptoms, such as numbness and tingling. This increases anxiety that results from these fears, which can result in hyperventilation, sweating, dizziness, chest pains, and other related symptoms. These people are now pretty sure that this constellation of symptoms is related to heart disease, which causes nervousness, which then increases the symptoms, and so on.

This cascade of events can lead to a full-blown anxiety attack or panic attack. Patients in this frame of mind often find themselves visiting an emergency room, visiting a doctor's office, or suffering silently on one's own. At the emergency room one would normally undergo cardiac monitoring, an EKG, and lab work, including cardiac enzymes (blood tests to see if there is potential heart muscle damage), which are often normal and usually unnecessary. One may or may not be admitted for further monitoring. On the other hand, they may be sent home before or after a stress test (that can also be done in an office setting). The costs associated with workups that are done due to underlying anxiety are certainly quite high, and would possibly not be needed if the underlying problem was resolved.

Ultimately, most are sent home after being told they suffered an anxiety/panic attack due to "just stress." Patients and doctors may misconceive that stress is not so serious, though this thinking shows a lack of recognition of how damaging stress can be to the body. They may be sent home with a minor tranquilizer, such as Xanax (alprazolam), Ativan (lorazepam), or another, and advised to follow up with their doctor. That person may follow up or just write the whole thing off as only the stress of the moment and think of it as "just one of those things." Some may obsess about it, due to the underlying anxiety, and get further workups by going from doctor to doctor, which is likely unnecessary and expensive.

If one does not go to the emergency room, but rather shows up in my office, I can assess whether or not they have an acute or more chronic problem and determine how much of a workup needs to be corrected to begin with. An EKG is easy enough to do and can be reassuring to both the patient and doctor. If I suspect an underlying cardiac problem, I would refer the patient to a cardiologist for further testing. Once I am reassured that the person's heart is fine, I can then concentrate on resolving the underlying anxiety causing these symptoms by balancing the nervous system. I have found that it is important to take the time to explain to my patients why these symptoms are occurring and what we can do about it. I explain the constellation of symptoms I previously described as being similar to a snowball rolling down a mountain. It can start small and get bigger and bigger as it rolls down the mountain, like the symptoms progressively worsening as the anxiety increases about the symptoms, which causes more symptoms and so on. This is yet another vicious cycle that thankfully can be broken.

If the symptoms occur more frequently when one is at rest, this suggests anxiety as the underlying reason and goes against the heart being the primary cause. If the heart were responsible for the symptoms then the symptoms would typically worsen with exertion and improve with rest. When a person is trying to relax, the stress that has built up in the body thus has an easier chance to come out, since the person's defenses are down and the person is more vulnerable. Stress-related symptoms are less likely to come out when a person is actively doing something, since the mind and body are active and preoccupied. I may remind patients that it is better to have these symptoms because of neurochemical imbalances, since they are easy to treat and not as immediately dangerous as having a bad heart. I also believe that adequate attention toward the prevention and treatment of mood imbalances in general would decrease the risk of heart disease.

The best thing to do when one has "cardiac symptoms" is to move the body. The tendency though is to do the opposite. One typically fears that too much exertion would over-stress the heart and make things worse. When fear and paranoia take over and interfere with reason, the mind can conjure up all sorts of possibilities. One's tendency may be to try to be as still as possible, which actually makes matters worse. Relaxation techniques can be helpful, and beta-blockers and other anti-arrhythmic agents can also be useful under certain circumstances when there is cardiac involvement. A beta-blocker also can work for performance anxiety, such as public speaking. Minor tranquilizers can be helpful for acute symptoms because they can quickly relieve the anxiety and related symptoms and potentially prevent an emergency room visit. The best approach, however, is to resolve the underlying imbalances in a preventative way with psychotropic medications, and thus be able to avoid the episode to begin with and decrease the need for symptomatic medications treating after the fact.

Metabolic Syndrome and Obesity

Metabolic syndrome is common and referred to by many names such as insulin-resistance, glucose intolerance, pre-diabetes, hypoglycemia, hyperglycemia, etc. This syndrome is caused primarily by genetics, but it can be exacerbated by poor lifestyle habits and potentially worsened by underlying neurochemical imbalances.

The main genetic defect that one develops is a resistance against one's own insulin, and the insulin thus does not function as it should. This can lead to increased sugar and carbohydrate cravings with a decreased ability to metabolize these foods. This can slow metabolism, decrease energy, and thus result in increased weight. Insulin resistance tends to cause an increase in abdominal girth in men and an increased size of the hips and buttocks in women. This can eventually lead to full-blown diabetes and increase the risk of heart disease and other medical problems.

Lifestyle changes are paramount, and I stress to my patients the importance of an exercise program and a well-balanced diet. Some have low motivation and low energy and are not willing, or able, to make these necessary changes. Some have obvious underlying mood disorders, such as depression, while in others it may be less obvious or not a factor at all. I have found that psychotropic medications can be very helpful for these situations since they can improve energy, motivation, drive, and metabolism. Certain medications combined in the right way can decrease hunger, decrease carbohydrate and sugar cravings, improve energy, motivation, drive, focus, and metabolism, such as Wellbutrin XL and/or Topamax, as well as a stimulant in some cases if needed and if tolerated. When mood and energy improve, it is more likely that one will eat better and exercise more often, which will result in feeling better and being healthier overall in the long term. This can lead to a dramatic improvement of one's quality and quantity of life.

ADDICTIONS
(DRUG ABUSE/ALCOHOL ABUSE/SMOKING AND OTHER ADDICTIONS)

Addictions can result when one attempts to medicate oneself. People abuse substances in order to "numb" themselves so they don't have to feel. Common addictions include drug abuse, alcohol abuse, smoking, excessive gambling, shopping addiction, sexual addiction, food addiction, eating disorders such as bulimia and anorexia nervosa, exercise addiction, internet addiction, gaming addiction, social media addiction, self-mutilation, and other behaviors that are taken to an extreme and unhealthy level. This results in imbalance in one's life which requires a course correction.

Common drugs that can be abused are prescription medications such as narcotics (Vicodin, Norco, OxyContin, etc.) and other pain pills, sedating muscle relaxants such as Soma, Tussionex and other codeine cough products, benzodiazepines (tranquilizers such as Xanax, Ativan, Klonopin (clonazepam), Valium, etc.), stimulants (Adderall, Ritalin and others, especially when not used for ADD), sleeping pills, and others. Some find it surprising that Vicodin and other narcotics/opiates are responsible for many rehab hospitalizations, as well as abuse of benzodiazepines and stimulants. This is because those who have an addictive personality may start out using them for a valid reason, but then take more and more if they are readily available because it makes them "feel" better. Addicts are "quick fix" thinkers who want to feel better *now*. This is why they prefer symptomatic over slower preventative medications that may take a week or two to see the full benefits.

It is disturbing that more people who are in rehab, or should be, are not taking psychotropic medications when needed. Some are told they should be "drug free," which unfortunately implies that they should also avoid preventative mood-normalizing medications. In my opinion, doctors and those in the rehab system and Twelve-Step programs (including sponsors) often do more harm than good if they promote this message. Those who believe this may find it more difficult to accept what I advise because they come to me misinformed. The spirit behind telling people to be "drug free" is admirable, but in practicality it is too broad a statement, and one that reveals the lack of understanding about this issue and the preventative and holistic nature of psychotropic medications. I therefore advise that those in rehab, or those who should be, to get their medical advice from someone who thoroughly understands this issue, and that would be a doctor that understands how to properly treat mind-body imbalances.

People who suffer from addictions are typically suspicious and hesitant about using psychotropic medications, even those who have not been misinformed by others. They may state that they want to improve their lives in a "natural" and "drug free" way because they fear trading one addiction for another. I explain that psychotropic medications are completely non-addictive unless feeling normal is an addiction, and it if is, so be it. These medications only help if there is an underlying imbalance that needs to be corrected. By using these medications, I have found that addicts will be more likely to stay away from the substances that they crave and abuse, and are less likely to relapse after recovery. This is because these medications provide a healthy way to balance the person's own neurochemistry and thus make them feel like their "old selves" again, which is even better than the way they felt with the use of addictive substances.

I have found that most people that suffer with addictions have underlying neurochemical imbalances that can be easily corrected. This makes a significant positive impact on their lives. If these imbalances are left untreated, they are much more likely to revert to previous unhealthy habits. This can potentially lead to a series of failed attempts at sobriety, which can further damage self-esteem and can leave them feeling more hopeless than they already feel. These people are at higher risk for a decreased life span and decreased quality of life in general. This vicious cycle can often be resolved very easily, safely, and effectively with the implementation of the preventative medication approach that I advocate.

Counseling is also important whether it be individual, in a group setting such as Twelve-Step meetings, or in a rehabilitation center. Some people do very well in a group environment which doubles as a support system, since others who have been there themselves understand what the person is going through. Many patients can learn better and healthier coping skills to help resolve the psychological components that lead to the addictions, which complement the treatment of the medical component with proper use of psychotropic medications. I try to be as encouraging and positive as possible in these situations, and I reassure them that going through this adversity can make them stronger in body, mind, and spirit.

Chronic Whatever

Pick a symptom, any symptom. If it is chronic, recurring, and otherwise unexplained, then assume there is a neurochemical imbalance somewhere behind that symptom and treat it as such until proven otherwise. Our index of suspicion should be high that there is a neurochemical link whenever a symptom or medical problem is either inadequately treated, is somewhat controlled but could be better, or when a problem is difficult to solve and one doesn't know how to go about treating it. There is nothing to lose and potentially a lot to gain using this trial-and-error diagnostic-treatment approach to ongoing conditions and complaints.

I can understand why some patients would be afraid to stop taking medications that ease their symptoms, but for myself, I tend to agree with those who are happy to get rid of the band-aids—that are not doing them a whole lot of good anyway—and get on with something that actually works on the problem and may even cure it, or at least control it.

Once patients and professionals in the health care industries grasp the significance of the role played by neurochemical imbalances as a primary cause of a host of physical and emotional conditions, the way treatment is administered will be forever changed. We will then see the next major turning point in the practice of medicine, and, as a result, our general view of life will be radically altered. The truth is that millions upon billions of people are suffering unnecessarily, and the help we need is right at our fingertips.

Chapter Nine

What Your Doctor Should Know (But May be Afraid to Ask)

We are now well down the road of the journey of discovery. Perhaps along the way your attention was drawn to something in particular. Maybe a description of a mood disorder or physical complaint sounds suspiciously familiar. You may find yourself wondering whether your symptoms might match a condition listed in the previous chapter. Or you may be thinking of a friend or family member whose bothersome emotional or physical complaints sounds like the very symptoms of one of those conditions. If so, you will appreciate this chapter, because it will prepare you for that potentially life-changing visit to the doctor's office. You are going to learn what you need to take with you to make the meeting as productive as possible.

Successfully treating an illness, injury, or disorder begins with a thorough knowledge of the problem. That thorough knowledge includes, not only your condition, but *you*. Whatever the nature of your affliction, it is attached to your body and is affected by your individual traits. You may say, "But what about a patient who is in a coma and cannot give the doctor information about herself?" Even then the doctor will ask friends and family questions that are vital to the treatment of the patient. For example, one of the critical questions to ask regarding a patient who cannot answer for herself is, "Is she allergic to any medications?" The doctor's knowledge of that one piece of information can make the difference between life and death.

So, if your doctor is going to treat you for a mood disorder or an undiagnosed chronic condition, you will have to provide information about yourself, your family history, and your previous experiences with symptoms, doctors, treatments, and results. This information is a necessary piece to the puzzle to help the doctor to prepare a workup and evaluation. Your doctor must be well-informed about you, and you are the foremost expert in the world regarding yourself.

You do not need to bring with you pages and pages of notes, but rather a summary. I can guarantee that your doctor will never read them or give you the chance to read them. Instead, I will show you how to streamline lists of the most important information so that you can quickly run through them with your doctor. Some physicians may be resistant at first, because they think you are going to take up too much of their time, but insist on being heard, and if you aren't go elsewhere. The truth is, though, that going through the important information up front will save a lot of time in the long run, because your concise report will enable your doctor to quickly separate primary issues from secondary ones.

Are Doctors Overworked?

Every doctor in the nation today feels the pressure of managed health care, excess paperwork, and working within the parameters of regulations, formularies, insurance forms, and countless other administrative issues. Many of them are also worried about the future of their profession, and for good reason. Doctors feel so beaten down by the inefficient and onerous system they are thrown into that many of them have lost their passion for medicine. In recent decades, since the very soul of medicine has changed, doctors who were trained to treat patients get frustrated when peripheral issues stand in their way. How can we provide adequate care for our patients if we have to squeeze them into five- to ten-minute appointments so that we have time for the hours of filling out forms that are waiting for us at the end of every day? Being pressured by the ticking of the clock, doctors tend to make quick decisions regarding diagnoses and treatment. Rushing and making decisions too quickly though is not the best way to address the proper balance of neurochemicals.

To provide the best care, family physicians must keep pace with the rapid change in several important fields, including general aspects of pediatrics, adult medicine, geriatrics, and gynecology. These are not easy subjects to master, and the information that the general practice doctor reads was prepared by specialists in their field and may require the physician's full concentration. Keeping up with all the issues of physical health care, many doctors simply feel like there is no time left over to deal with psychiatry/mental health, so they prefer to refer patients out to professional counselors or psychiatrists if they detect a mood disorder or psychosomatic illness.

As we have seen, the most common problems that create distress and pain for people are not *psych* problems, but rather the real medical problems of neurochemical imbalances. If doctors would *make time* to learn how mood-normalizing medications resolve many of the problems that people bring to the office every day and if they would *make time* to go over the patient's history, they could radically reduce the incidence and severity of many other medical problems. When doctors begin to address these neurochemical issues, they will be saving themselves time and saving time, money, and needless suffering for their patients. We have every reason to work at achieving this win-win situation.

YOUR INITIAL VISIT

There are three important issues you need to bring to your doctor's attention during the initial visit. If there is not enough time to address each one, plan on covering more during your next visit. If necessary, little by little you will get through to your doctor and begin to look like a person and not merely a problem.

The important issues to address are:

1. A detailed description of symptoms.
2. A detailed past medical and medication history.
3. A detailed family history in order to pinpoint genetic causes.

Each item provides clues about your condition and offers insight on how to proceed. Learning how to treat individual patients is a process, so your doctor will be asking questions about peripheral issues along the way. Do the best you can on your side of the conversation, because good results begin with good communication and honesty.

When you go into the office for your initial consultation, remember that the most important diagnostic tools are the doctor's ears. Listening to your history provides your physician the basis for making the best diagnostic decisions. So make certain you bring with you a detailed description of symptoms, including past symptoms, current symptoms, and how they may have changed over time. Your symptoms are clues as to which neurochemical(s) are most likely to be imbalanced, which then guides the physician to make the best treatment decisions.

There Are No Irrelevant Symptoms

There is no single symptom or set of symptoms that are specific to a neurological chemical imbalance. As we saw in the previous chapter, the conditions that cause mood disorders can also cause physical pain and undue stress on the body's bones, muscles, tissues, skin, and organs. I am quite certain that there are not only patients, but also a good number of doctors who will be surprised to discover all the symptoms that can be traced back to an imbalance within the nervous system.

For that reason, it is important that you prepare a complete list of your recurrent symptoms before your first visit. Even if you think you know the cause of some of your symptoms, assume that chemicals also play a role until proven otherwise. This way your doctor will not miss any vital information that may mean little to you, but be very significant to a health professional.

Few people really grasp how much the various pressures of life create stress that takes a toll, not only on our emotions but also on our bodies. For that reason, we take a painkiller or muscle relaxant when we have knotted muscles in our shoulders and neck or suffer from a tension headache. We do not appreciate why our back "goes out" every time we go through a stressful or sorrowful life event. We do not listen to our bodies when they are trying to make us conscious of an internal problem.

Most of us know when we are in pain or when a lump or bruise appears on our body. When we find a dark mole with an irregular shape that we do not remember seeing before, we may think to ourselves, "I should have that checked." If we put this off, we soon forget about it and discover that even little aches and pains can be easily ignored. We do not realize that dismissing these things and the subtle changes in our body or mood can have serious consequences, because the minor symptoms are connected to glands and organs where the problems become critical. I am not saying run off to the doctor with every little joint pain, but when you make the list of symptoms for your doctor to review, include everything we have discussed to this point.

As a general rule, the higher the number of symptoms, the greater the likelihood is that they stem from a neurochemical imbalance. The same is true of the number of symptomatic medications one takes (band-aid type medications that relieve symptoms rather than solve problems).

PERSONAL HISTORY

The next important part of your initial evaluation is a personal history. Make certain that you disclose to your doctor as many details as you can remember whether or not you feel they are pertinent.

Where to begin your personal history: Go back in your memory to the last point in your life when you felt your very best in mind and body. We always begin here, because our goal is to recover that same level of health and happiness. From there, work your way forward to the present. As you come to significant changes, your doctor may be able to see a correlation between an age-related hormonal change and the onset of a mood disorder, for example. If you remember never feeling quite the same after a particularly difficult illness, this will alert the doctor to chemical changes your body may have undergone due to the sickness. As a matter of fact, simply reading this book and becoming familiar with the types of things that can produce a chemical imbalance and how that, in turn, can result in unpleasant symptoms, will enable you to recognize potential imbalances on your own. Do not be afraid to suggest to your doctor what you have concluded about your condition. Better that you say it and risk being corrected than to keep it to yourself and go on believing the wrong thing about your health or even doing something that may compromise it.

What to include in your personal history: Include every major event in your life, like losing someone close to you through death or divorce, major moves, serious illnesses, or any other major stressors. By the way, even good events can still be very stressful, because adjusting to them places demands on our mind and body that our nervous system must accommodate. Looking back over the changes in your life—some for the better and others for the worse—is helpful information if it is pertinent, because it is easier for you and your doctor to determine where to go when you know where you have been.

FAMILY HISTORY

Finally, your family history is vital to your doctor. Be concise when you write out the history, because you want to cover as many factors as possible. For example, if your list includes information like, "My father went through a ten-year depression, attempted suicide once, and was hospitalized for three months," this will give your doctor vital information. Keep your descriptions short and let your doctor ask you questions if more information is needed.

Heredity is the most common cause of neurochemical imbalances. You have inherited genes from both your parents, who inherited their genes from both their parents, and so on. Sometimes the physical and mental history of an uncle or aunt can be as significant as that of your mom or dad. You get more of a "genetic load" from parents and relatives you resemble most with regard to looks and personality. Do not underestimate the importance of providing the doctor with an accurate and complete family history. I am sure that you can appreciate the significance of your genetic background, because genes are commonly linked to many medical problems, including high cholesterol, hypertension, heart disease, diabetes, low thyroid, mood disorders, alcoholism, chronic pain disorders, etc.

In general, when genes play a significant role in chemical imbalances, the symptoms tend to be more severe and more difficult to treat. A history of neurochemical imbalances on both sides of your family puts you at greater risk than if only your father or only your mother or either side of the family had shown symptoms of the imbalance. I say, "shown symptoms," because it is likely that if your parents, and especially your grandparents, had a chemical imbalance it was never diagnosed, since much less was known about this then as compared to now.

In the "old days" of American history, most people did not admit to any sort of emotional weakness. Instead, they just bore it and avoided open discussion of personal problems since they did not want to look like they were "crazy" or weak. There were also myths of stoic resignation or the idea that it was noble to suffer and to keep it to yourself. As a result, there was a lot of silent suffering. (By the way, those modes of thinking sound a lot like current day thinking for the majority of people.)

Here are a few clues to help you and your doctor uncover neurochemical imbalances that may run in your family:

1. History of alcoholism and/or drug abuse

2. History of violence and/or abuse

3. Flawed core parenting skills

4. Chronic and recurring pain associated with symptoms

5. Parents that were very moody and "snapped" easily, were nervous, depressed and other such hints that there was a mood disorder or chronic recurring physical symptoms that may hint toward underlying chemical imbalances within the nervous system as the true underlying cause.

Mood disorders and other evidence of neurochemical imbalances can be tracked in the details of your family's history. As I tell my patients, "You can change the jeans *on* your body, but not the genes *in* your body." Fortunately, though, the good news is that in our modern era, the negative results due to those genes that leave you predisposed to a chemical imbalance can be altered through mood-normalizing medications and compensate for what genetics has denied you.

CONCLUSION

After obtaining information about your symptoms, medical, medication, personal, and family histories, your doctor is ready to make an educated guess as to which medication or combination of medications will address the neurochemicals that are suspect. We may not get it perfectly right the first time, but the rational trial-and-error process will most likely eventually produce the desired results.

For this reason, your doctor will hopefully prescribe one medication or another after your first visit. You will want to know what the medication does and what your doctor is hoping to accomplish. Also inquire as to what options you have for backup medications if the first trial does not work. Whether it works or not depends on your report at the follow-up visit. How you feel, whether you have experienced relief, and whether there are significant side effects is all important information to convey.

The most important aspect of the doctor-patient relationship is honest and thorough communication. If there are barriers that prevent communication, then we must work together to break them down and establish mutual trust. The more we work together, the better we will be able to determine the best course of action. As long as the communication lines are open, we can make corrections as we go and in this way come to a scientific conclusion through learning by experiment and experience.

Again I want to remind you that medications are not the only treatment option. At the risk of sounding like a broken record, regular exercise, a well balanced diet, psychological counseling when needed, relaxation techniques, prayer and meditation, all serve to enhance our quality of life. When we treat the body right, there is a lot of healing and self-correcting that it can do on its own without medications. When our body hits the wall, then the next step in holistic health is to assist it by balancing its neurochemistry with mood normalizing medications.

We are on the same team, working together to reach the same goal: Your optimal health and well-being. The more we can remove the stigma of mood disorders, decrease cynicism toward people who offer substantial help, and reduce the hesitancy people have about seeking help, the more healthy and happy people we will encounter. Why would we want anything less for ourselves or our family and friends? We begin with as simple a step as patients and doctors learning to communicate and cooperate with each other. Taking this approach to the practice of medicine, I have found my patients to be my best teachers and my favorite works of art.

HEALING
— THE —
MIND AND BODY
VOLUME 1
SECOND EDITION

— SECTION IV —

DEPRESSION, BIPOLAR DISORDER, AND EATING DISORDERS

- THE D-WORD
- THE UPS AND DOWNS OF BIPOLAR DISORDER
- EATEN ALIVE BY EATING DISORDERS

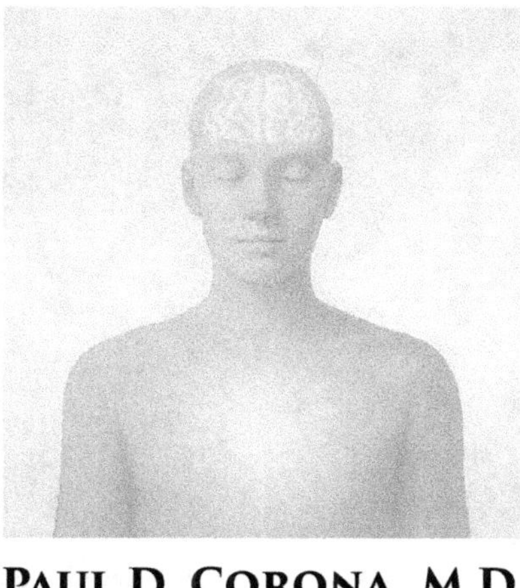

PAUL D. CORONA, M.D.

CHAPTER TEN

THE D-WORD

In case you have not guessed, the "D-word" is depression; a subject few people care to discuss. Some people are afraid of depression, as if it were a black hole whose gravity is so great that not even friends or family can avoid getting sucked into it. Other people have an aversion to depression because they equate it with defeatism, a weak self-image, lack of will power, the sissy's response to life's challenges. Still others have found it to be a strange and mysterious disease that can suddenly invade any person's life and then stubbornly refuse to leave. We avoid the D-word, fearing that we give it an existence by merely saying it or that by pronouncing the word we conjure the dark spirit.

Personally, I am not particularly fond of the word depression, and that is why I refer to it as the D-word. My discomfort with the word depression is not only the negative bias it creates in our thinking as soon as it is spoken (much like the emotional reaction of a patient who hears the word "cancer"), but because people attach so many different meanings to the word that it has become fairly useless as a diagnostic term. Some people think that depression is merely choosing to see "the glass half empty." Others think the depressed person is wallowing in self-pity or is merely an old grouch. Still others believe one is depressed when one cannot eat or leave the house, but cries all the time and talks about suicide, which is actually a severe clinical depression, though this is the least common type.

If we are compassionate, we pity people in depression. If we are totally ignorant regarding depression, we blame the victim. If he would simply "look at the bright side" or if she would "make a list of all the things she had to be thankful for," he or she could quickly snap out of it. Optimistic and relatively normal people do not know the gnawing pain of living for years with a brain that is constantly drowning in despair. But the optimist is equally a mystery to the depressive who cannot fathom how a person is able to find hope for the future, their family, their work, or anything else.

During a consultation two years ago, a woman was describing the horrible pain she felt in the grief of losing her mother to cancer. She said that sometimes it was so intense that she felt like she was suffocating, like she could not survive another day of it. I let her go on for as long as she needed to express her anguish. Then, when she finished, I said, "This is a miserable and hopeless feeling, isn't it?" "Oh yes," she answered, "I've never felt anything this awful before." I then said, "This is what some depressed people feel nearly every single day of their lives." At first she looked slightly bewildered, then shocked. "That must be terrible. I can't imagine a fate worse than that." I assured her that I would make sure she would not feel that way for long.

We are going to pull back the curtain on depression and learn not only something about its causes, but also its cures. Before we conclude the chapter we will also review anxiety disorders, ADD/ ADHD, and Obsessive-Compulsive Disorder (OCD). If you think that you do not have OCD because you are not one of those people who have to wash their hands a hundred times a day, you are likely to benefit from learning something about the varied and milder cases that can make a normal life unnecessarily difficult and unpleasant.

The Rising Cost of Life in the Twenty-First Century

Consider the number of stress-producing experiences that happen in a week and that we have come to accept as a normal part of life: a child comes home with low marks on a report card, the car needs an expensive repair, a marriage begins to show signs of disintegrating, food and gasoline prices rise while our income remains static, our new supervisor turns out to be a total jerk, we are transferred to another state, our child is found in possession of marijuana, and the list goes on and on from neighbors whose dog is a pest to a government that has grown so large that it cannot keep track of its own body parts yet must keep feeding itself, to prevent going on a much-needed diet.

Add to these stressors the factors we have covered in previous chapters, such as genetics, hormonal changes, illnesses, a weakened immune system from too much stress for too long, drug and alcohol abuse, and the typical traumas of life. We also have to take into consideration the nutritional deficit of a typical American diet, the feeling of being too hurried to take time for proper exercise, lack of a spiritual connection for many, and lack of attention to one's health in general. Is it any wonder that mood disorders are on the rise due to the body's chemical balance being thrown off by one or more of these conditions of our everyday lives?

The Myth of More

Frank strolled into our office because he heard through the grapevine that I was successfully working with a variety of antidepressants. Suffering from depression, he hoped that I could help him achieve a heightened sense of well being. Before he came to see me, he had done his homework and read up on depression and its roots in the brain's neurochemistry. During our appointment, he confidently anticipated a regimen of medications that would boost the levels of serotonin and dopamine in his brain. Frank had been taken in by The Myth of More.

When people first learn that there are chemicals in the brain that promote good feelings, they have the same reaction as the medical community did in the infancy of the neuroscience of mood disorders. They jump to the conclusion that their suffering is the result of an inadequate supply of the right chemicals and assume that medications are used in order to increase the production and supply of the chemicals. Their thinking, in fact, is like that of people who use drugs recreationally to give their mood a lift. Some of the early attempts to medicate depression were based on the same assumption.

Since those early days, however, research in the field of neuroscience has uncovered the fact that the brain of a normal, healthy person has no problem producing serotonin, dopamine, and so on. The problem is that, even though these chemicals are already present in the brain, and that a person has the right amount, they are not doing their job. For some reason, they are not moving from one neuron to another, as we saw in an earlier chapter. In other words, the problem is not due to a chemical deficit, but a chemical imbalance.

The medications we use to balance neurochemicals do not add active chemicals to the circulatory or nervous systems. Instead, by attaching to the nerve cells, these medications allow the brain to put to good use the chemicals that are already present in the synapses between neurons, but need help moving along. They have been designed by pharmaceutical companies to address specific neurochemicals in specific ways to produce the proper and healthy balance. Balancing neurochemicals is effective only if an imbalance was at the root of the patient's disorder in the first place. These medications do not automatically make people feel better—they are not "happy pills" as patient's sometimes refer to them, or "happiness in a bottle." Rather, if needed they can lead to true underlying natural happiness.

The challenge faced by doctor and patient is to determine as clear a diagnosis as possible to predict which neurochemicals are imbalanced and to what degree. Then a medication or a combination of medications are prescribed to correct the specific imbalances. The medications enable the nervous system to do its job by removing the roadblocks and fixing the leaks. As I often explain to patients, it's not up to you or me to decide which medication or treatment plan is right for you, but rather it is up to your body.

The body has an amazing ability to heal itself when it is functioning normally. The doctor's humble role is to listen to what the patient and the patient's body have to say about the potential imbalances and then do as the body dictates. For the benefit of the body, the doctor will administer the smallest amount of medication possible to complete the job if done correctly. Thankfully, doctors improve their diagnostic skills over time, as we acquire knowledge by listening to what the patient and the patient's body have to tell us.

Response and Remission

When we treat a mood disorder or psychosomatic condition, what are we hoping to achieve? In the medical community, the words we use to describe our goals are recovery, response, and remission, while at the same time working to prevent relapse and recurrence. Researchers in the fields of mental and physical health try to put a specific value to these terms so that patients and doctors have some kind of tool to rate the patient's response to treatment, whether their condition is improving, worsening, or staying the same.

For example, in dealing specifically with depression, one of the most widely used rating system for research purposes is the Hamilton Rating Scale for Depression (HAM-D). The severity of one's depression is determined by the answers one provides to a clinical interview. Each answer is assigned a numerical value and when the numbers are added up, a doctor or therapist will determine whether treatment is called for, and if so what level of treatment. Generally, patients will be interviewed again after a few weeks and months of therapy or medication to determine their progress. There are other rating systems for a variety of mood disorders and psychosomatic conditions

(MADRS, HAM-A, LSAS, YBOCS, PANSS, ACDS, etcetera, etcetera).

Now suppose a patient suffering from depression has a HAM-D score of 30 on a scale of 0-50 on their initial visit, which means they definitely need treatment. Like in golf, the lower the score the better. Let's say that after a month of medication and talk therapy their score drops to 15. We have seen a fifty percent improvement in their condition, which indicates a "response" to the treatment they are receiving. The government requires pharmaceutical companies to conduct tests that indicate their product can produce this baseline result (fifty percent) in order to win approval for sale and distribution.

Most people in the throes of depression would be thrilled to experience a fifty percent improvement and most doctors would be happy to see their patients make that kind of progress. In fact, on the surface, a fifty percent advance toward better health and happiness is a worthy accomplishment. That is, unless a one hundred percent improvement is possible. Who would settle for feeling half as good as they are capable of feeling? This is the mind-set we should have regarding the treatment of chemical imbalances: Fifty percent improvement is good, but not good enough if a higher percent is easily within reach. A HAM-D of 7 or less has been one of many definitions of full remission. My goal for every patient is a HAM-D score of zero, or at least as close as possible.

Hopefully it is clear that I am not satisfied if my patients merely respond to treatment. Rather, I want them to experience full remission. If a patient does not experience full remission, we should assume that the mind and body are still working apart. Remission is the gold standard when evaluating the effectiveness of our use of medications. Full remission is achieved when patients either feel like they are back to their old selves again or perhaps feel even better than they have ever felt in their lives. Our first goal is to get to full remission as quickly and as safely as possible. Our second goal is to keep patients there for the rest of their lives.

We use the word recovery when remission lasts for six to twelve months. Relapse is a failure to maintain remission or if the condition worsens. Recurrence indicates that the patient enjoyed a period of recovery, but eventually fell back into the previous condition. There are many reasons for a recurrence of depression and they are usually not the patient's fault. However, sometimes patients will do something (discontinue their medication on their own because they feel better) or not do something (seek help through talk therapy, eat right, exercise regularly, or withhold important information from their doctors) that contributes to recurrence.

We use the term full remission when the patient's symptoms of depression disappear completely. Those in full remission discover a new patience, presence of mind, and calmness in handling the difficult issues of life, feeling stronger from within, and back to their old selves (or even better). They are no longer irritated or upset by the things that used to disturb them. Patients sometimes wonder how these "drugs" I am prescribing them resolve so many issues in their life and give them a sense of empowerment when facing mental and physical challenges. I have to explain to them that the "medications" are not controlling their thinking or feelings, but are putting them in control of their bodies and moods.

As we discovered in an earlier chapter, optimum health and well being is greatly affected by the doctor-patient relationship. For this reason, we need to be in agreement regarding our goal for the patient's improvement. A doctor who hopes for no more than a positive response to a medication can undermine a patient's healing who is hoping for full remission. Rather, a patient who is satisfied with fifty percent improvement, or at least as close to that as possible as "good enough" may hold their treatment at that level and frustrate the doctor's attempts to achieve one hundred percent improvement. A person who has experienced years of depression can find it difficult to believe that full remission is possible, but let's agree on having that as our target and, together, do our best to hit that mark or at least get as close as possible.

A Critical Question for Establishing Our Goal

There is a question that I ask my patients during their first visit and initial evaluation: "Looking back at your life from childhood on, at what point do you remember feeling your best? What age were you when you last felt truly happy and positive about life?" The most common answer is, "That would probably have been when I was in my early to mid-twenties." If not their twenties, most patients will say, "When I was a child until about ten to twelve-years old." (Assuming it was a happy and healthy childhood, free of abuse, neglect and significant trauma.) Other slightly less common answers are the teenage years and the thirties. There is nothing surprising about these answers, because it correlates with a pre-adolescent state of physical stability prior to puberty in which significant genetic and hormonal changes occur.

Those earlier times of well being are remembered as a life that was simple, carefree, fun, and free of all the stress and worry that came later. As we mature, we accrue greater responsibility. Life becomes more complicated and stressful, and many of us lose our youthful optimism not to mention other life enhancing pleasures, like our sense of wonder, free imagination, and love for learning. Because these changes occur gradually, we hardly notice how much they affect our mental or physical health, and if we do notice, we merely chalk it up to aging. We do not realize that we do not have to live with increased anxiety, a decline in mental outlook, or a host of aches and pains.

The question regarding patients' earlier time of happiness and the answers they give are critical in establishing two fundamental considerations for treatment: First, they give us a benchmark for setting our goal. We need to have in mind a specific idea of what it is we are trying to accomplish or recover. Some patients find it difficult to believe that it is possible for them to recover their "old self" of an earlier time in life when they were happy and relatively stress free. Our goal is to restore that level of well being or at the very least get them as close as possible.

Secondly, the answer to this question is frequently a good indicator in diagnosing the neurochemicals that need to be adjusted. If we can connect the onset of a mood disorder to a significant life-change in their past, then we have a clue to how that event affected their neurochemistry. As humans age (from birth to death), they constantly transition through developmental phases which are generally preceded by hormonal changes. Some of the better known and more radical transitions include maturing into adolescence, early adulthood, mid-life, and the later stages of life. Women have the additional possibility of significant hormonal and chemical changes of pregnancy, the postpartum period, and menopause (and some researches have started to address "male menopause"). There are also other "events," such as illness, injury and stroke, that can produce chemical changes that affect a downturn in the patient's mood.

A patient whose childhood was so dysfunctional that they cannot remember ever feeling happy or positive about life, along with a patient who has suffered memory loss due to a head trauma, will require special care. However, it is still possible, and I believe necessary, to establish a benchmark for wellness, and in these radical instances of an unhappy life or a lost memory of happiness, we create the target of "feeling better than you have ever felt before or even dreamed possible."

TREATING DEPRESSION

The sad and melancholy mood disorder known as depression is as old as recorded history, celebrated in poems and romanticized in the suicides of famous people. For the person who suffers depression, there is nothing festive or romantic about it.

Common features of depression include:

- Recurring sadness
- Crying easily
- Irritability
- Decreased interest in activities that a person had once enjoyed
- Insomnia

- Fatigue
- Feelings of worthlessness
- Feelings of hopelessness
- Feelings of helplessness
- Decreased ability to concentrate
- Recurring thoughts of death
- Recurring worry
- Recurring guilt
- Obsessive tendencies
- Recurring pain and other recurring somatic (physical) symptoms

Depression has a high level of recurrence, which means that for many sufferers it never goes away completely, even on their good days. For others, depression is so pervasive they cannot imagine what it would feel like to have a "good day."

Once we bring depressed patients to full remission, how long should they continue to take their medications? The question seems like a simple one, but the answer is surprisingly difficult.

Some people would assume that medications are no longer necessary once their depression goes away, while others would assume that they will have to be on medications the rest of their lives. However, the actual situation with any patient will vary anywhere from one end of the spectrum to the other. Some patients merely need to work through a difficult season of their lives or a sudden avalanche of overwhelming misery as in post-traumatic stress disorder, while others have always been depressive. If the neurochemical imbalance is the result of an acute event such as death of a spouse, divorce, loss of job, or sudden illness and has not been a longstanding problem, then the course of treatment would usually be short-term. However, if the condition has been chronic, involves greater stress factors, and has a stronger genetic load, the patient will more likely remain on a long-term regimen. In every case though, it is up to the patient's body to decide when to adjust a dosage up or down or go off of a medication altogether.

My objective is to begin to reduce and discontinue medications as soon as possible, once we have some kind of indication that there is not a likely chance for recurrence. The current rule of practice is to cut back or discontinue medications after the patient has enjoyed at least six months of full remission and then monitor their progress. However, I have found that at least an entire year of full remission is generally a better time frame, because it gives the patient time to receive talk therapy and begin to form new thinking habits to break the pattern of their old depressive rumination. If depression recurs, it would then be reasonable to resume medications for at least two or three more years. If there is another recurrence after that cycle, then the patient will probably need life-long treatment. Keep in mind that these are very rough guidelines that are affected by the chemistry, personality and specific needs of each individual.

When patients discover they will have to take medication for the rest of their lives, I say, “So what”? Conditions that require ongoing medications are quite common, including diabetes, hypothyroidism, arthritis, and so on. Lots of people suffer from asthma attacks, allergies, and seizures. Everyone gets sick at some point in their lives and, in my opinion, everyone should be immunized against polio, diphtheria, tetanus, measles, mumps, and other debilitating or life-threatening diseases. The great thing about mood normalizing medications is that they are nontoxic and can be taken for a lifetime without doing any organ or tissue damage.

If, however, a patient experiences unwanted side effects from a particular mood normalizing medication and discovers she will have to be on meds for a long time, she and her doctor will need to determine how to proceed. For example, if the side effects are minor and if the improvement is significant, the patient may choose to put up with the side effects, which may resolve over time. If the side effects are too uncomfortable or annoying to tolerate, the doctor and patient can usually find other medications that will work as well without producing the same side effects. Sometimes swapping medications or adding a medication to reduce side effects actually results in an even greater improvement, so there is no good reason to avoid experimentation in these cases.

RECOMMENDED MEDICATIONS AS A FIRST RESPONSE:

- An SNRI (one of the 4), usually at a low to moderate dose.
- An SSRI can be a good agent if norepinephrine does not need adjustment, otherwise balancing norepinephrine and serotonin are important when physical symptoms and anxiety coexist with depression.
- Wellbutrin (bupropion) is also recommended as an augmenting agent to adjust dopamine. It may be used as a solo agent, but is more likely useful when added to an SNRI or SSRI in order to both reduce side effects and improve overall results.
- Lamictal (lamotrigine) is recommended if depression is the downside of a bipolar disorder.
- "Atypical" antipsychotic medications are very useful for "treatment-resistant" depression, bipolar depression, and other more difficult-to-treat variations of depression. Lithium and other mood stabilizers also are useful for resistant depression with suicidal ideation.

- Deplin (L-methylfolate), Nuvigil (armodafinil)/Provigil (modafinil), stimulants and other augmenting agents (such as a thyroid supplement for hypothyroidism or a testosterone supplement for hypogonadism) can be effective for some people.

Treating Disorders Related to Depression

Anxiety Disorders

Life-threatening situations, extremely unfortunate events, and demanding decisions or activities, will normally produce anxiety and trigger the autonomic nervous system into the familiar "fight or flight" response. Anxiety becomes a problem when it persists over time, intensifies without being aggravated by any circumstantial cause, or interferes with a person's everyday life. Anxiety disorders are characterized by some or all of the following symptoms:

- Persistent or recurring symptoms such as restlessness and agitation
- Difficulty with focus and concentration
- Irritability
- Insomnia
- Muscle tension
- Sweating
- Elevated heart rate or blood pressure

- Hyperventilation/shortness of breath
- Dizziness
- Fatigue
- Somatic symptoms with chronic and recurring pain syndromes
- Excessive worry

Depression and anxiety are not easy to separate, because they share common causes, effects, and symptoms. Patients who are depressed and patients with anxiety disorders will typically spend a lot of time ruminating over their circumstances, past events, and potentially bleak futures. Both conditions involve some sense of inadequacy and play on the patients' fear. In both cases, a chemical imbalance is a contributing factor and frequently the treatment for one will work effectively for the other.

I have had patients ask me, "Why did you give me an antidepressant? I'm not depressed. I'm just stressed out." There is rarely such thing as a pure form of a mood disorder, but rather conditions and symptoms overlap, people respond differently to the same neurochemical imbalances, and the whole human psyche is simply way too complex to reduce to a textbook diagram.

Anxiety disorders, like depression, entail what I call the "lettered" disorders, because so many acronyms have been coined to describe them. Some items on the following list will probably be familiar to you:

1. SAD (social anxiety disorder)
2. PTSD (post-traumatic stress disorder)
3. GAD (generalized anxiety disorder)
4. MDD (major depressive disorder)
5. OCD (obsessive-compulsive disorder)
6. ADD/ADHD (attention deficit disorder with or without hyperactivity)
7. PMS/PMDD (premenstrual syndrome)

The letters are not important, because what matters is whether any of these conditions are affecting a person's quality of life. It is less important to know what causes the anxiety, but rather that the anxiety exists and interferes with normal functioning. The definitions can be useful to indicate a chemical imbalance, but we need to avoid the illusion that sometimes arises when we can label a condition. The illusion is that a label tells us all we need to know about the person and how to proceed with treatment. Humans cannot be reduced to neat and tidy categories and will not respond well to treatment that is based on rigid, outdated, and incomplete guidelines. To achieve the best results with anxiety disorders we have to be willing to think outside the box and not latch onto only the "approved" medications determined by the FDA or insurance companies.

Anxiety is characterized by a wide variety of symptoms and, therefore, usually requires the combination of different medications to address all the needed adjustments. Neurochemicals to address in the following order:

- Norepinephrine (especially when physical symptoms are also present)
- Serotonin
- Dopamine and GABA are also often involved.

The general rule is that more than one neurochemical is involved, which usually requires a combination of medications in order to achieve the best results.

Recommended Medications Include:

- An SNRI
- An SSRI
- An "Atypical" (Dopamine balancing) agent should be considered when anxiety is linked with a subtle variation of bipolar disorder.
- Topamax (topiramate), Neurontin (gabapentin), Depakote (divalproex sodium), Lyrica (pregabalin) or Trileptal (oxcarbazepine) can be useful as GABA balancing agents when the nervous system requires that it be stabilized.
- Medications to treat sleep disorders related to anxiety may also be prescribed.
- Tranquilizers can be useful for acute anxiety symptoms, but their proper role should be on an as-needed basis only.

I feel it is absolutely necessary for me to remind you that any and all of these medications should be started at the smallest dosages that are most helpful with little or no side effects for the optimal length of time. I have found that combining medications has proven most effective in the treatment of anxiety disorders. If doctors and patients make one mistake too often in this regard, it is the leap to unnecessarily high dosages, which can create or exacerbate other problems. However, high doses are best for some cases, so we need to individualize treatment.

Obsessive-Compulsive Disorder (OCD)

OCD covers a constellation of disorders. The classical presentations are well recognized: frequent and numerous instances of hand washing; checking and rechecking things such as houselights, locks, and appliances; repeating a behavior a specific number of times; and saying certain numbers or words over and over again. These are the more extreme presentations and are easy to recognize, but there are far more subtle presentations of OCD, such as excessive rumination, not being able to let go of a task even when it is inane or unnecessary, overworking, and having difficulty falling asleep because the mind simply will not "shut off." The purpose of OCD-related behavior is to provide a coping mechanism that appeases patients' anxiety and calms their worry. One symptom sometimes seen in OCD is that patients realize their actions do not make sense, yet they cannot stop. They are haunted by the fear that failure to engage in a repetitive or ritualistic behavior will result in some sort of misfortune or painful consequence. Their fear also leads them into a self-perpetuating cycle of obsessive thinking. OCD is not uncommon in any of the addictive behaviors that control people and keep them bound to behaviors long after they are no longer enjoyable or even desired. Addiction behaviors with such things as drugs and alcohol, smoking, gambling, shopping, sexual fantasies and encounters, eating disorders, overexercising or excessive attention to one's appearance are employed to give the OCD sufferer a temporary relief from anxiety and depression.

Serotonin is the classic chemical implicated as being imbalanced in OCD, though the other neurochemicals can also be involved. As with the other disorders, I have found that most likely more than one neurochemical is involved.

Recommended Medications:

- An SSRI is the classic medication class to use for "classic" variations of OCD, and usually higher than average doses are needed. Luvox (fluvoxamine) is the most specific SSRI indicated for OCD, though the other SSRIs also work.

- If the classic case is not resolved with an SSRI, then other chemicals besides serotonin should be addressed.

- Agents to balance norepinephrine as well as serotonin and the other neurochemicals are effective for patients who suffer other disorders with OCD such as anxiety or somatic disorders.

- Anafranil (clomipramine) is a tricyclic antidepressant (works on serotonin and norepinephrine) that can be useful for more resistant cases of OCD that don't resolve adequately with other more first-line agents.

Attention Deficit Disorder (ADD)/ Attention Deficit Disorder with Hyperactivity (ADHD)

ADD, in my opinion, can be either underdiagnosed or overdiagnosed. The actual incidence of ADD has more to do with the way people think and process information rather than a deficiency in their thinking ability. For example, we frequently hear that children who have ADD have difficulty with concentration or the performance of necessary or sequential tasks. However, if you watch the average boy who has been diagnosed with ADD play a video game for hours, you realize there is no problem with his concentration, recognition and organization of information, or sequential processing to solve problems and carry out a task when he enjoys what he is doing.

The challenge of ADD is not so much attention as it is attraction. If a person with ADD is not attracted to a topic, task, or assignment, he finds it impossible or nearly impossible to focus his attention. This is what results in the high distractibility associated with ADD and the tendency to focus intense concentration on the "wrong" things. For example, after class, a student with ADD may be able to give an accurate and precise report on what a teacher was wearing and not remember a word of what she was saying.

People with ADD have difficulty progressing through a rigid system where memorization and performance of specific tasks is rewarded, while free thinking and exploring different ways of solving a problem than those presented are punished. There are people in industries that are beginning to appreciate the value of "ADD thinking" and making room for the free range of a mind that does not do well when it comes to playing by the rules.

However, ADD is a problem for those people who think in this different way, because it is unpredictable and can interfere with critical decisions and actions when a procedure or specific order of steps must be followed. ADD also interferes with education because it takes the student's focus away from the subject at hand. As a result of doing poorly in school, people with ADD are frequently ill-equipped to handle even some of the simple and important tasks in life, like filling out a job application or even balancing a checkbook. They are overwhelmed by all the possible ways they could answer a simple question on a form, such as, "Give the name and address of your last place of employment." The answer seems simple enough to the applicant who knows what the personnel supervisor is asking, but the person with ADD is bombarded with a dozen different possible answers and feels he must guess at which answer will satisfy the supervisor.

Those with ADD can struggle over something so simple as filling out a form during the first visit in a doctor's office, creating for themselves a lot of unnecessary fear and anxiety. Sometimes a doctor can quickly identify this person, because when he shows up for his appointment, it is his wife who came with him that talks with the receptionist, carries the insurance information, and fills out the forms.

ADD can surface as early as preschool to kindergarten, but for most children it becomes more noticeable when their academic demands increase in the third or fourth grades. Children with ADD who are also hyperactive are more easily diagnosed at an earlier age, whereas children who are introverted may be able to hide it until a later age. However, most cases of ADD do not include a discernible excess of hyperactivity, so we need to be alert to the possible variations of this disorder.

Because of the complications ADD creates in a person's ability to move normally through the education system—the first experience of an institutional environment that most people with ADD encounter—they often develop other mood disorders, such as depression and/or anxiety (this is referred to as comorbidity when one disorder is accompanied by another, which is very common with ADD). This is because they are constantly made to feel stupid or like a failure, being constantly reminded of their shortcomings by the circled, red "D's" and "F's" on the top of many assignments. Many students eventually internalize the "F' and it becomes a defining factor in their self-perception. Not surprising, estimates of prison inmates who have ADD are as high as eighty percent (only fifty percent were actually diagnosed with ADD when they were children). They almost all also have other comorbid conditions, with a particularly high incidence of bipolar disorder.

Both ADD and comorbid conditions are related to neurochemical imbalances, and patients who are diagnosed with these conditions can benefit from mood normalizing medications, stimulants, or a combination of both. If treated at all, ADD is most often treated with stimulants like Adderall (dextroamphetamine-amphetamine), Concerta (methylphenidate hydrochloride ER), Ritilan (methylphenidate), as well as several other medications that are amphetamine-based. The stimulant medications for ADD do not deserve the bad reputation given to them by the overexposure of an uneducated media. True, some people have abused these medications and that possibility is always present. Doctors, as best they can, must monitor their patients' use of every medication they prescribe as well as those prescribed by other doctors. Parents also need to monitor their children's use of medications, and, in most cases, parents should have the medications in their possession and dispense it daily as required.

The most common side effects produced by stimulants are activation (over-excitation of the nervous system), fatigue, decreased appetite with accompanying weight loss, insomnia, apathy (not caring, lack of motivation), flattening of the personality, elevated blood pressure, and very rare cardiac risks. Obviously, patients need to be examined by their physician before a stimulant is prescribed. Generally, the side effects of stimulants occur only when the dosage is too high, if it is the wrong medication, or if it needs to be combined and balanced with non-stimulant medications.

Some patients find that when their chemicals are properly balanced by mood-normalizing medications, they no longer need the stimulants. Others experience the best results when mood normalizing medications are combined with stimulants, which can result in the patient's thinking being the clearest and most focused.

ADD is still a relatively new diagnosis, and there are a lot of questions about it that remain to be answered. Sometimes ADD diminishes and even disappears on its own as the person matures. Many people adapt their job situation around it. For example, an executive may have his or her secretary organize and manage their time.

If symptoms of ADD begin to appear in adolescence, but were not a factor earlier in the child's history, I have found that this usually signals chemical imbalances due to hormonal changes during or after puberty, which is not actually true ADD, but rather one of the comorbid conditions mentioned. I occasionally see some diagnosis with "adult ADD" that is not really ADD, but rather ADD-like. True ADD usually starts in early childhood. However, the diagnosis sometimes becomes more obvious in adulthood, as it's presentation earlier in life may be subtle, unrecognized and thus untreated for years due to the patient's natural high intelligence.

In these cases, after a thorough history and physical, the teenager or adult can sometimes be treated with a balanced diet, hopefully a somewhat balanced lifestyle, and mood normalizing medications if there is an underlying mood component, which I have found to be very safe and effective in these age groups. Even if non-stimulants improve the symptoms of ADD/ADHD, stimulants are still often very helpful for most people who have ADD/ADHD.

Some psychologists use written tests to diagnose ADD and other specialists advocate a differential diagnosis (distinguishing one condition from another) based on medical, oral, physical, and written tests, by a panel of experts. In my own practice I take a thorough history, and then I use a trial period of one medication at a time to determine if ADD is present or whether something else is interfering with the patient's thinking, or if it is a case of ADD with comorbidity.

If the results of our tests prove to be as good as, or better, without using a stimulant, that is my preference, although stimulants have often produced excellent results in controlling ADD, and have been considered the "gold standard" treatment. It's really not my nor the patient's preference that is important, but rather the preference of the mind and body of the patient.

Other medications I have used are:

- An SNRI can also work as an alternative to stimulants, or in addition to stimulants. If the patient has somatic symptoms along with symptoms of anxiety, depression and/or ADD all at one time, an SNRI would be an ideal choice.

- Wellbutrin (bupropion IR) can be used as a solo agent or combined with other medications by inhibiting the reuptake mostly of dopamine and some of norepinephrine.

- The SNRI-Wellbutrin XL combination balances serotonin, norepinephrine and dopamine at the same time, the original "Dynamic Duo."

- Strattera (atomoxetine), (an NRI-Norepinephrine reuptake inhibitor) in place of stimulants or, in some cases, with stimulants.

- Provigil (modafinil)/Nuvigil (armodafinil) is a non-stimulant that boosts histamine and dopamine, that has been shown to be helpful for some patients.

- Stimulants quickly move the neurochemicals forward and also slightly inhibit the reuptake of dopamine and norepinephrine.

- An "Atypical," a GABA agent or other mood stabilizers can also be helpful for some if bipolar disorders coexist with ADD, which is not uncommon and can be challenging to treat.

Some may feel uncomfortable that I advocate the use of medications, such as mood-normalizing medications and stimulants, for children. I have found them to be extremely safe and effective when prescribed properly. I don't feel comfortable discriminating against people who need medical help based on age. I am an advocate of reducing human suffering whenever possible, and the children who grow up hating themselves and thinking of themselves as worthless or dumb because they perform poorly in their early education, need and deserve our assistance. This can damage one's self-esteem and confidence at a very vulnerable time in one's life, and can prevent the real underlying full potential of an individual from becoming realized. What a waste. Also, the risk of addiction is much higher if it is not treated.

There is also another benefit that often accompanies resolving a child's ADD. Since ADD definitely indicates a genetic link, when a parent sees their child's remarkable improvement through the proper balance of neurochemicals, they frequently ask if there is something that the adults in the family who have ADD can take that will work as effectively. They may now want to do as well and feel as good as their children and adolescents do. In those times, I have the privilege of helping entire families by walking people out of a lifetime of haze into a new world of clarity. The practice of medicine cannot get much better than performing this kind of service for individuals and their families, which also benefits society as a whole.

Chapter Eleven

The Ups and Downs of Bipolar Disorder

I had settled into my flight to Chicago, where I was registered to attend a conference on Bipolar Disorder. To be honest, I have generally used speaker training conferences like this to catch up on some much-needed rest, reading, and writing without having to manage the constant demands of the office. Not that bipolar disorder was unimportant to me, but I was thinking, "Yeah, I know about this condition, they used to call it manic depression, but it's basically the same thing." What a shock when I sat through the first seminar and heard statistics and insights that I had never read in any journal or textbook, and I found myself furiously taking notes. I could not ditch the seminars for recreation and rest, because I was fascinated by the new revelations uncovered in recent research regarding this prevalent and sinister condition. During the plane ride home, I organized my notes and wrote what would later be the basis for writing this chapter.

Bipolar disorder has become a topic I love to write and speak about because it is both interesting and extremely important, not to mention that it is much more common than the healthcare community had realized. When the facts surrounding this disorder are fully known, its recognition, diagnosis, and treatment are going to have a profound effect on society as well as individual sufferers.

Bipolar disorder is grossly misunderstood and misdiagnosed. By some estimates, it is ten times more common than patients and doctors realize. The main reason for the confusion and general ignorance about bipolarity is that it presents itself in more than one form. Only the most radical variation, Bipolar I, has received any significant attention in the media. Bipolar I affects about one percent of the population, however the reality is by my estimation that more than ten percent of the population has some variation of bipolar disorder. I think this estimate is very conservative since, in my opinion, it is even higher. The suicide rate for bipolar disorder is much higher as compared to unipolar disorder, so it is also the most dangerous mood disorder of them all.

When you read in the paper or hear in the news that someone who has been known as a fairly normal person suddenly, and without reason, went off the deep end and committed some bizarre crime, committed suicide, or other irrational act,

Bipolar I is generally at the root of their behavior. People who have Bipolar I are likely to think irrationally and act impulsively, e.g., frequently gambling for high stakes and shopping sprees in which they purchase items on credit they cannot afford. Many of them are risk-takers, engaging in extreme sports or driving dangerously on public streets and highways. During this stage of Bipolar I the erratic behavior of the patient sometimes resembles psychosis (schizophrenia). In other words, the person suffers a serious break with reality. I have referred to bipolar disorder as "schizophrenia-lite," since they share certain features that may not present as extreme or persistent. There can also be confusion about the distinction between ADD and bipolar disorder, although there are ways to distinguish between the two. They also can coexist, which can make treatment more challenging.

Unfortunately, the insane behavior of certain high profile crimes committed by people with this strain of bipolarity has caused some observers to ridicule or trivialize the reality of this condition, the magnitude of its impact on a human life, and the desperate need we have to help these people for their sakes and for ours. There have been other sufferers who have performed acts of great heroics and self-sacrifice while quietly bearing the torture of this condition in solitude. Bipolar I, however, is at the extreme end of a continuum of less serious strains that are much more common, yet personally devastating, and also potentially life threatening.

BIPOLAR AND UNIPOLAR

If you know the difference between a bicycle and a unicycle, then you can guess at the difference between bipolar and unipolar. A bicycle has two wheels and a unicycle has only one wheel. "Polar" refers to an axis (imagine a straight line that runs from one point to another) that stretches from one pole to another, as illustrated in the phrase, "They are poles apart."

Bipolar Disorders — Unipolar Disorders

Clinical depression is an example of a unipolar disorder, because the patient experiences one mood disorder and only one. Other examples of unipolar disorder were covered in the previous chapter. The bipolar patient also knows depression, but can also make radical swings into mania—a state of elation, agitation, and possibly paranoid and psychotic thinking, in which a person's racing thoughts make it difficult to sleep or exercise sound judgment.

The term rapid cycling is used to describe the frequent jumps from one pole to the other that some patients experience, four times per year or more in some cases. A mixed state occurs when a patient experiences mania and depression at the same time. These variants can be the most challenging forms of bipolarity to treat.

Bipolar II disorder is distinguished from Bipolar I because the manic phase is less extreme. The standard definition of Bipolar II is depression with hypomania (that is to say, "mild mania" or what I refer to as "mania-lite"), and it affects two to three percent of the population. This less severe form of bipolarity is still a serious disorder, accompanied by anxiety that is more intense than unipolar anxiety disorder, and depression that can cycle and get deep and dark at times. Remember that most of bipolar disorder is spent in depression, not mania or hypomania. It can also manifest some of the same symptoms of the more severe bipolarity: racing thoughts, agitation, and insomnia.

The type of bipolarity that is most widespread among the general population is currently labeled Bipolar NOS (Not Otherwise Specified), and is sort of a catchall for the many variations that do not fit into the other two classes. Cyclothymic disorder is characterized by both hypomania and hypo-depression (dysthymia), referred to as cyclothymia. There are many other lower grade forms of bipolar disorder that express in many different ways. The most subtle variations are most often recognized as difficult-to-treat unipolar disorder, such as "treatment-resistant depression." (I have found that "treatment-resistant" usually means one is treating the wrong diagnosis in the wrong way).

Bipolar NOS in all its variations affects sixty to seventy percent of those suffering with bipolar disorder, and possibly more because people whose mood swings are not extreme are less likely to seek therapy. Therefore, the statistics are likely to rise as the research into bipolarity becomes more refined and as it is recognized and reported by more people in the healthcare profession. We know two things for certain at this time. First, the list of conditions that fall into the bipolar category is continuing to grow. In addition to Bipolar 1 and 2, there is also Bipolar 3, 4, 5, and 6, with subtypes, and more to come. Second, in the not too distant future, many people will recognize themselves in this growing list and will not have to live with the symptoms of their own suffering.

Detection

Bipolar disorder is commonly misdiagnosed as one of the unipolar disorders. I have found that is especially true regarding anxiety. One of the most common misdiagnoses is failure to distinguish the anxiety of unipolar disorder from the hypomania of bipolar disorder. When bipolarity is misdiagnosed as one of the unipolar disorders, doctors have a difficult time resolving the condition and frequently refer to these cases as treatment-resistant, such as treatment-resistant anxiety or treatment-resistant depression. Some physicians substitute the word chronic for treatment-resistant, because the condition keeps recurring or, more likely, never goes completely away, but merely cycles to the other pole for a while. Bipolar disorders, though, are resistant to treatment only when it is not recognized for what it is and treated accordingly.

The dramatic and radical presentations of Bipolar I or II are certainly fascinating, and bipolar patients in the manic phase can be energetic and a lot of fun, but this is only temporary. However, there are more subtle versions of the disorder, and they present greater challenges for the doctor who needs to determine what is at the heart of the problem as quickly as possible. It is very important to keep in mind that usually much more time is spent in depression than in mania and patients more likely seek help when depressed, while when manic they are out having "fun" and don't want a doctor to slow them down. This is why taking a detailed history is so important to see if mood cycling occurs over time, looking for depression, hypomania and mania, and how often these cycles occur.

I do not mean to frighten you with this next bit of information—though I have to admit I personally find it very disturbing—but it takes an average of four psychiatrists between seven to ten years before they can, with certainty, diagnose bipolar disorder. Not taking a thorough history and not understanding the full spectrum of bipolar disorder are some of the reasons why.

I have found that working with people who have the milder versions of bipolarity are just as fascinating to treat as the more extreme cases. Challenging? Yes, absolutely. However, it's also interesting as the doctor works as an investigator following the clues, and it's exciting when the right medications are prescribed and patients recover their lives.

Turning Over Rocks (or Diagnosing Bipolar Disorder)

Like every other disorder, bipolarity manifests symptoms, and by tracking those symptoms we can find our way to the cause. I do not mean to imply that this endeavor is easy, but I simply want to emphasize the fact that we can learn to recognize many features of bipolar disorder. These features and symptoms provide us with the clues we need for a diagnosis and treatment strategy.

Family History

The family histories of bipolar patients are more "loaded" with instances of troubled and unstable relatives than their unipolar counterparts. There have been times when, having suspected a bipolar condition, I asked the patient if any other family members have a mood disorder, to which the patient responded, "How much time do you have?" or "Let me tell you about my family!" In fact, it is not unusual for a bipolar patient to report mood disorders in family members of both parents, which is less likely the case with unipolar patients.

Unipolar patients tend to present milder stories of their family background and are, therefore, less likely to have chemical imbalances as severe as bipolar patients. The more genetically similar a person is to the family members that had the most severe imbalances, the more likely that person will have a similar disorder. In summary, genetics is not to be overlooked when one is evaluating mood disorders since this information is of vital importance.

Drug Abuse

There are a staggering number of people with bipolar disorder who abuse drugs—well over fifty percent of all bipolarity cases. The fact that these people would be inclined to self-medicate regardless of legal, mental, physical, and relational risks is hardly surprising. Depression, the downside of bipolarity, is so dark and miserable that the need for even a temporary and synthetic relief is difficult to resist. Some bipolar people look for their lift in soft stimulants, such as caffeine, "power drinks," or weight-loss products like those found at health food stores (so-called "metabolic enhancers" that may include ephedrine or (ephedra-like) substitutes, which may pose serious risks, such as hypertension, seizures, heart attacks, and strokes). Others jump right into the hard stimulants, cocaine, speed, and methamphetamines.

At the other end of the pole, the upside—manic, anxious, agitated—are people who long for a moment of peace and calm, more than three hours of sleep per night, and something to "calm their nerves." These people turn to drugs that help them relax: Alcohol, smoking (THC as well as nicotine), prescription tranquilizers (Xanax (alprazolam), Valium (diazepam), Ativan (lorazepam), Klonopin (clonazepam), etc.), sleeping pills, muscle relaxants, opiates, and nonprescription drugs including herbal remedies. Patients with bipolar disorder typically take higher doses of tranquilizers and sleeping pills more frequently than those with unipolar disorder. However, none of these substances are true remedies, because they merely treat symptoms and do nothing to address the underlying cause.

I am going to throw out a teaser here and develop it more later on. There are two parts to what I have to say and the first part should be no surprise: People who are controlled by addiction to drugs or alcohol can be helped significantly in the recovery and sobriety phases by adjusting their neurochemistry until it is balanced. Unfortunately, the organization that has had the greatest success in helping people recover, Alcoholics Anonymous (AA), is biased against almost every kind of pill that affects moods. Their reticence to getting hooked on painkillers or tranquilizers is completely understandable, but not enough people in AA realize that mood normalizing medications are not mood enhancing (in the sense that they produce a false or chemical high). The second part of the teaser is this: When working with someone who has self-medicated with soft or hard drugs, *the patient's drug of choice is a significant indicator as to which medication or medications are likely to be most effective in resolving their condition.*

Mood Instability

The psychologically correct term is Mood Lability, and refers to a constantly changing or unbalanced emotional state. A labile condition can be observed in someone who fluctuates from a positive state to a negative state, who is excessively emotional (laughing too hard and long or constantly weepy), or who is both up and down at the same time (e.g., an "energetic" and "active" type of depression, perhaps smiling on the outside while extremely depressed within). Their families describe them as "up and down" and cannot predict what sort of mood they will be in from one day to the next—although this is generally an exaggeration because, in most instances, one mood persists for several days.

Living with someone who has this condition is like riding an emotional roller coaster. The person may be easily angered, turn on a friend or family member without warning, prone to start fights, or go through life perpetually irritable. They are sometimes prone to injury and compound their problems through high-risk behaviors and poor judgment, such as indiscriminate sexual activities. This is because they tend to be impulsive, not think through the consequences, and frequently act on a whim. Bipolar patients who are subject to these mood swings may do something that they later regret when they swing out of the mania phase. In fact, they not only calm down, but their emotions and energy can descend into the darkness of depression and self-loathing. Sometimes there are external reminders of their erratic behavior—an injury, a damaged relationship with a loved one, or court appearances and legal actions. In those moments they will ask themselves, "What have I done?" or "What was I thinking?" Guilt and shame are likely to drive them deeper into depression, which may spring back later on into even more radical stunts. There are some bipolar patients who are also sociopaths, and they do not feel any regret or shame and have no conscience. In fact, they feel nothing in regard to the trouble, damage, or pain they have caused.

Social Anxiety

Social anxiety—extreme shyness, quirkiness, and awkward behavior around others—is more typical of unipolar disorder, but it is sometimes present in bipolarity. Those who are bipolar are usually the shy people who seem "a little different" or "just a bit off" and display more irrational thinking or behavior. The majority of these folks keep to themselves and avoid harming others, while inside their own minds they experience silent torture. But in the most extreme cases, their social maladjustment causes them to hate other people, to devise plans of hurting others, and can potentially "snap." That is when those usually quiet, depressed, and shy people surprise everyone who knows them in some outrageous act of striking out at the world by brutalizing or killing innocent victims.

CHAOTIC LIFESTYLES

Bipolarity creates not only a restive spirit, but it makes a normal, ordered, and predictable life nearly impossible. For that reason, people with this condition tend to move and switch jobs frequently, have difficulty sustaining any sort of responsibility that requires regularity in emotional, relational, and physical stability, and go in and out of marriages. Statistically, bipolar disorder accounts for a higher rate of infidelity and, on average, a history of multiple sexual partners, which is due to their addictive personalities. Therefore, they are more prone to sexually transmitted diseases, may spend their spare time in strip clubs, and have a higher risk of obsession with pornography. These behaviors may be related to the manic or hypomanic state, whereas during the depressive state they may show little interest in sex.

The inability to form lasting relationships or be present to others results in trouble at home, school, work, and with friends. Bipolarity is not only likely to get a person fired, but it also interferes with landing a new job because getting a decent referral from a former employer is not easy. Recognizing and treating these patients appropriately will lead to a more productive work force and to more stability with relationships and life in general.

Personality Disorders

Every healthcare professional who has worked with bipolar patients knows very well that these people are likely to have other character disorders. Doctors can use this information to their advantage when diagnosing bipolarity, because, along with other symptoms of this condition, they can make a note of the fact that their patient is overly dramatic (histrionic), narcissistic, has what is referred to as a "borderline" personality disorder, or some other excessive personality traits.

Due to their personality disorders, these patients tend to be difficult to get along with and are avoided in social environments—others may perceive them as different or weird. Doctors and their staffs are not particularly excited to see them either. Initially they may be too friendly, but sooner or later they often become unpleasant and noncompliant. When they visit their doctor, they are more needy, annoying, or upsetting than other patients. Unfortunately, for all the good that mood normalizing medications can do, they cannot change a person's core personality, though they can tend to decrease the excessiveness. Psychotropic medications can take away the "rough edges" and extreme nature of the imbalanced personality, making it easier and more likely to change.

Character disorders are sometimes evident by the obnoxious way the person treats other people (an exception would be the sociopath who can be quite charming until it is time for them to strike, then they injure others without a twinge of regret). When bipolarity is suspected along with a personality disorder, indications to look for would include whether the patient is excessively talkative or loud, talks too fast and stumbles over their words (since their minds go faster than the words come out), and a lack of consideration for others.

The average person without extensive psychological and medical training and tools is wise to avoid developing too close a relationship with these people. Those rare people who realize that they have a personality disorder and want to change or adjust to a normal life have been able to make excellent progress through extensive therapy. However, the road they take to get there is not easy.

SENSITIVITY TO ANTIDEPRESSANTS

Bipolar patients sometimes have a surprisingly quick response to antidepressant medications, showing improvement in record time. This fact in itself is a tip-off for the doctor to keep an eye out for other indications of bipolarity. When the correct antidepressant is prescribed, the bipolar patient will usually show optimum response at a dosage lower than that of an average unipolar patient. The same is true of the unwanted negative side effects of an antidepressant in that there is a higher sensitivity to potential side effects at lower doses.

Because these patients tend to be hypersexual, they may refuse to take medications that will potentially affect their libido. If a patient seems overly concerned about the sexual side effects of a medication before agreeing to take it, the doctor should red flag their comments and be alert to any other signs of bipolarity. Unipolar patients share a similar concern but to a lesser extent.

Some people with bipolar disorder have learned to exploit their manic phases, and the way they can work during this part of the cycle makes it seem like they have superpowers compared to other workers. When they have used their mania energy to succeed, they are skeptical of medications that might make them lose their "edge." These people are not dummies. In fact, they are normally quite intelligent, usually more than those without bipolar disorder. Intelligence though does not always provide the same benefits as wisdom which, if listened to, will prevent people from crashing emotionally and physically by chemically leveling their mood and pacing themselves for the long run.

Since bipolarity can cause a person to be easily distracted and impulsive, doctors must be careful to distinguish it from ADD, because the primary treatment for ADD can worsen the symptoms of bipolar disorder and push a patient into a full-blown manic episode. Stimulants prescribed for ADD can cause a bipolar patient to suffer insomnia and loss of appetite, agitation, and worsening of mood. There are alternative treatments that may be safer for those with addictive personalities, those who cannot tolerate stimulants, or those who are at higher risk for drug abuse or relapse if exposed to a stimulant. For those with bipolar disorder and ADD, a stimulant with adequate mood stabilizing with other medications can be safe and effective for most patients who have this combination.

Insomnia

A detailed sleep history can be an invaluable guide in helping to diagnose bipolar disorder. We will want to hear the patient's answers to the following questions:

1) Do you need less sleep than others you know?

2) Is your mind racing so fast at night that you can't keep up with it at times?

If the patient responds to the first question with something like, "I don't need a lot of sleep. Three or four hours of shut-eye and I'm good to go" and to the second question, "How did you know? Every night my brain just won't shut off. My thoughts spin out of control and I can't get to sleep." Answers like these strongly hint at bipolar disorder.

During the manic cycle of bipolarity, many patients find that staying up late into the night is their favorite time for getting things done. To compensate for lost sleep, some will take naps during the day, but many merely skimp on sleep.

During the depression cycle, they may find themselves waking up between two and four o'clock in the morning, feeling miserable, desperately wanting to fall back to sleep, but unable to do so. Because they are hypersensitive to any kind of stimuli, they are easily awakened by noise, hunger, thirst, and even a small amount of fluid in the bladder can make them feel like they have to get up several times during the night to use the restroom.

Restoring normal sleep cycles is one of the significant milestones in addressing bipolar disorder, and this can usually be accomplished by adjusting the neurochemicals until they are properly balanced. As simple as it may seem, just getting enough high quality sleep can make a huge difference in how the bipolar patient feels. As a rule, medications that balance dopamine (the "atypicals") or GABA prove to be the most effective agents for producing deep, restful and refreshing sleep.

A Quick Buck

Some of these patients get involved with "get rich quick" schemes. They can be easily duped by others who talk them into getting involved with various kinds of schemes and scams. In spite of their intelligence, they do not manage money well—or their lives, for that matter. They will invest in high risk ventures and then berate themselves when they lose their investment. This can also cause a lot of marital and family stress as well.

High Achievers

The super energy of the manic cycle of bi-polarity has given rise to some renowned works of art, literature, music, architecture, and business. No wonder many of them would be happy to eliminate the depressive cycle, but hate the idea of losing the mania. For that reason alone many of them will resist taking medications. In my experience though, balancing chemicals to level out the bipolar patient does not in any way compromise the quality or creativity of their work. What they do not realize is that they are sacrificing a lifetime of excellent work for a short, but active, period of work at a great cost to their health, relationships, and stability in life.

Psychosomatic Complaints

Chronic headaches, abdominal pain, pulled muscles, and so forth are not unusual in cases of bipolar disorder. Psychosomatic complaints are more common with unipolar patients, but it is the bipolar patients who are the most melodramatic when they describe their symptoms. If a doctor suspects that the patient's overreaction to their symptoms may be one of several indications of bipolarity, the theory can be tested by prescribing medications that address serotonin, norepinephrine, or even better, both at the same time. When given these meds, if the patient does not quickly show signs of improvement or doesn't tolerate them, the doctor has one more indication of bipolar disorder.

Grandiose Thinking

Because a bipolar person in the manic phase can work circles around everyone else—the normal people who need sleep, work reasonable hours, and enjoy spending time with their families—they tend to think of themselves as superior to others. They may become bored or easily frustrated when they have to work with people who, in their view, are beneath them. They are often very demanding and assume that they are entitled to extra attention and special treatment. They may call doctors by their first names and treat the office staff like their servants.

Some of these patients are name-droppers and besides exaggerating their number of friends, they also fudge their knowledge, skill level, and actual accomplishments. They frequently complicate their lives and those around them by the number of fabrications they invent. The world of their bipolarity is so chaotic and difficult that it seems they must invent a more pleasant life or image of themselves where they are more like a superhero than a broken human.

Treatment: The Rational Polypharmacy

I want to spell out what I mean by rational polypharmacy. My method of applying mood normalizing medications is that of polypharmacy (poly, "more than one"), because I emphasize the point that different medications at carefully adjusted dosages can be combined in certain ways to treat the various disorders covered in this book. My approach is rational in that it involves a systematic approach of an educated understanding of neurochemistry and how to achieve a properly balanced nervous system (rather than the complete guesswork of shooting in the dark). Rational polypharmacy progresses in the following way:

1. The doctor conducts an extensive evaluation of the patient.

2. One medication is prescribed at a low dose, and it is then best to taper it up slowly as needed and as tolerated. It just depends on the particular needs of each individual. This medication serves two purposes: First, to begin to resolve the patient's imbalance, and second, to confirm that the doctor and patient are addressing at least one of the neurochemicals that needs balancing.

3. The doctor and patient discuss and evaluate the change or changes the patient experiences with the first medication, paying close attention to all the details provided by the patient. The next step they take depends on their assessment of the patient's progress.

4. If the initial results are positive, but not completely satisfactory, the doctor will have enough information to tweak the diagnosis and narrow the search for the specific neurochemicals to target. At this point the doctor and patient can either switch to a different medication or add a medication to more effectively address the imbalances.

5. Poor results or significant side effects of the initial phase of medication also provide the doctor with excellent diagnostic information. Knowing what does not work is an important clue to knowing what is more likely to work. If a medication is ineffective, you conclude, "One neurochemical down, three to go."

6. A medication that results in slight improvement may be prescribed at a higher dose. All the while it is important for the doctor and patient to maintain a high level of confidence that they are on the right track, that they are learning more with each phase, and that they will find the right combination of

meds at the right dosage to bring the patient to full remission or, at the least, to a much more improved state than their current condition.

The rational polypharmacy approach is important to understand, because it is the best treatment strategy for patients with bipolar disorder, as well as all of the other variations of neurochemical imbalances. The many variations of bipolar disorder and the unique ways that it affects each individual requires an intelligent and closely monitored program. As we will see next, these patients will show the greatest improvement when they are taking a combination of different medications at low to medium doses. The key advantage to the rational polypharmacy method is that we minimize negative factors and maximize the beneficial properties of the medications.

Getting Started

Most doctors believe that the best first-line medication to use in treating bipolar disorder is a mood stabilizer, and the "classic" mood stabilizers are Lithium Carbonate and Depakote (divalproex sodium). These medications can be effective for some patients, especially for those who have Bipolar I disorder. However, they can also pose certain problems for patients. Lithium Carbonate does not work as quickly for mania as Depakote or the atypicals and also requires periodic blood monitoring.

Lithium Carbonate is known to cause unacceptable side effects for some, such as fatigue, dizziness, and weight gain. Depakote works quickly for mania, but also requires periodic blood monitoring and can cause fatigue, weight gain, and hirsutism (abnormal hair growth) in females, etc. I have had good results for some patients with these agents, but overall I view them as second- or third-line agents since we now have other medications available that are potentially better and have less severe side effects.

My first-line treatment of bipolar disorder comes as a surprise to many people, because the most effective medications are those that were originally developed to treat schizophrenia. These medications are known as atypical antipsychotic medications, and they help to keep the mind grounded in reality. However, as I made clear in an earlier chapter, some of the most effective uses of mood normalizing medications cannot be found on the label of the prescription bottle or the package insert or the medication handout the pharmacist can provide, which is more confusing than helpful. These medications have more uses than what the pharmaceutical companies are allowed to print, so the discovery of "off-label" benefits of a medication is extremely fortunate for bipolar patients.

Recommended medications include:

- Abilify (aripiprazole), Geodon (ziprasidone), Risperdal (risperidone), Seroquel (quetiapine),

Invega (paliperidone), Zyprexa (olanzapine), Saphris (asenapine), Latuda (lurasidone), Rexulti (brexpiprazole), Vraylar (cariprazine) and others, with more to come. These medications do not usually require blood monitoring, and, in general, they are well tolerated.

- When these medications are prescribed at their most effective dosage, they may cause daytime drowsiness. Therefore, the addition of a low dose of Wellbutrin (bupropion IR) to a primary agent often quickly resolves these side effects. However, the doctor and patient must be alert to the possibility of triggering hypomania or mania by the addition of Wellbutrin, which I have found to be an invaluable medication.

- An antidepressant added at the right time is very effective for most bipolar patients. However, prescribing antidepressants to bipolar patients is controversial for fear that they may induce mania. I agree that doctors should proceed with caution when treating Bipolar I disorder, especially for someone who indicates rapid cycling or more intense phases of mania. However, since this type of bipolarity is very rare, we should concentrate on the subtler variants of the condition that we encounter more frequently.

For a patient with a history of mania or hypomania, but comes to the doctor in an acute state of depression, it is reasonable to start an antidepressant before a mood stabilizer. However, we must watch closely to prevent triggering mania. If the depression resolves quickly without serious indications of mania, then it is most likely safe to continue the antidepressant while we quickly add a mood stabilizer. However, if the depression begins to resolve, but the patient becomes unstable, I would stop the antidepressant, quickly stabilize the mood and then reevaluate adding an antidepressant at the appropriate time.

- For patients that do not have a significant history of depression, a mood stabilizer may be sufficient. However, to achieve full remission with most patients, the addition of an antidepressant will be necessary.

- Balancing GABA sometimes helps as either the sole mood stabilizer or in combination with another medication. This class would include Depakote or Topamax (a weaker stabilizer, but sometimes more effective in milder cases), Neurontin (gabapentin), Trileptal (oxcarbazepine) and Lamictal (which really doesn't increase GABA, but rather inhibits glutamate). Lamictal (lamotrigine) is an excellent antidepressant choice for bipolar disorder, either Bipolar 1, Bipolar 2 or more subtle variations, with cyclical depression, for those who don't tolerate the "classic" antidepressants, or for more chronic and difficult-to-treat depression.

If both poles of bipolar disorder—i.e., mania and depression—are not fully treated, the patient will not experience full remission. Since mania has proven to be a dangerous state, the temptation is to focus on that side of the disorder rather than depression or the other physical and emotional symptoms that stand in the way of achieving the best results. Suicides are not uncommon during the manic phase, but more common during the crash into depression that follows.

The most common side effects of the atypical antipsychotic medications that I recommend include:

1. Weight Gain

These medications inhibit the release of dopamine, which can increase hunger and food cravings. If a patient gives in to those cravings, which usually include carbohydrates and sugars from unhealthy sources, they will gain weight. This is manageable though so long as the patient pursues a healthy lifestyle, regular exercise, and a well-balanced diet. Another way to manage food cravings is to add a medication such as Topamax, Wellbutrin, a stimulant or other weight loss medication. Some antipsychotic meds result in weight gain more than others. If this is the case, an alternative medication in the same class of atypicals may resolve it, such as Latuda, Saphris, Geodon, Vraylar, ones that are potentially more "metabolically friendly." Then again there are some bipolar patients who have a high metabolism (due to the mania phase) or a decreased appetite (especially during the depressive state) and cannot maintain a healthy weight. For them some weight gain may be an advantage.

2. Glucose Intolerance

This side effect has been exaggerated in the media, primarily by lawyers who promote unnecessary fear in order to generate more clients. Unfortunately, patients with bipolar disorder have an increased risk of diabetes compared to the average population and are, thus, more prone to glucose intolerance even when not on "atypical" medications. If a person was susceptible to diabetes and weight gain specifically in regard to an atypical, then we would have a problem. However, all medication interventions require us to weigh the positives and negatives for each patient. Glucose can always be monitored in the office and even at home if it is a concern. If it should arise as an issue, the treatment can always be changed. Keep in mind though that when a person feels well and healthy they are more likely to keep themselves in that condition, and the better the nervous system functions the greater a person's health will be overall. In most cases by far, the gains outweigh the risks.

3. Sedation

Some atypicals have a greater tendency to cause drowsiness than others. However, even this is often an advantage rather than a disadvantage since insomnia and anxiety are prominent features of bipolar disorder. If fatigue carries over into the daytime, I would decrease the dose of medication, change medications, or add a medication to combat sleepiness. Augmenting agents like Wellbutrin (most commonly), an SNRI, a stimulant and Provigil (modafinil)/Nuvigil (armodafinil) can not only reduce side effects but frequently bring about an even greater improvement in the patient's well-being.

If a patient is acutely manic, the doctor will begin with a high dose of a medication to resolve the condition as quickly as possible. However, seeing bipolar patients in this state is very rare in a clinical setting, and therefore dosages should usually begin low and gradually be increased and augmented until the desired effects are achieved. In this way, we can be certain that we are treating the patient with as low a dose as possible, while maximizing the benefits of the medication to the individual.

Maintaining Control

After a patient's bipolarity is under control, the next challenge is to keep it under control. Bipolar patients tend to be impulsive, to make decisions on their own, and frequently take themselves off of their meds when they start to feel better. If a patient experiences fatigue, he may decide to take himself off of the mood stabilizer. If he no longer feels depressed or thinks the antidepressant is affecting his sex life, he may stop taking it. Sometimes these patients think they can figure out what they need on their own, so they increase or decrease the dosages without consulting their doctors.

Bipolar disorder requires treatment at both poles of the continuum, so the medications and dosages may need to be switched and changed when they cycle from one mood to the other. Patients can be taught ways to discern the onset of mania or depression—and families can be especially helpful in this regard—and encouraged to contact their doctor if ever they have any concern that they may be cycling. Bipolar patients are also notorious for needing ongoing adjustments to their medications as they age, so their relationship with their doctors is a crucial factor in maintaining the good health they achieve.

The good news is that bipolar disorder can be managed, resolved, and in most instances treated to full remission. People do not need to live with this stubborn, disturbing, and life-threatening condition. We need to get the word out regarding how many people suffer needlessly with this condition that is vastly underdiagnosed and undertreated, and explain how an educated application of some new and remarkable medications can help them discover what normal feels like, and how wonderful life can be when their moods are not jerking them upward and then slamming them back down.

This book is my attempt to let you and others know how your world can be turned right-side-up so that you can rise to the top of your game.

Chapter Twelve

Eaten Alive By Eating Disorders

Ellen wanted to be loved. Actually, there were many things she wanted, mostly the things that everyone desires out of life—to be noticed, liked, educated, employed, married, cared for, and have an opportunity to serve others. A belief though had been programmed into Ellen's mind, so deep she was not even aware that it was there, and for her, that belief had become reality: No one would ever find her attractive, love her, want her, marry her, and there was nothing she could do to change that sad fact.

Overweight as a child, Ellen's father constantly teased her about being fat, and it made no difference in her adult life whether he had made his remarks to her playfully and affectionately or in mean cruelty, because either way they had done irreparable damage to her internal world. By the time she reached puberty in junior high school and, like all adolescents, had become self-conscious, the cutting remarks of other kids combined with her awkwardness in physical education and exclusion from most social events, Ellen's destiny was all but sealed.

Even if Ellen had attended a school where the students were kind or had grown up around gentler human beings, she would have still developed a sense of gross inadequacy or unacceptability based on teen magazines that target young women. The images of near-skeletal models and articles about how to lose weight to be more attractive to boys, how to know if a boy likes you, and how far you should go on your first date, would have been a constant reminder that she was simply the wrong body type. Therefore, for most of her early life, Ellen felt doomed.

When Ellen moved into her room in the college dorm, she nearly despaired when she met her roommate, a slight coed with twig-like arms and legs the thickness of a pipe cleaner. Rachel immediately accepted Ellen, was super friendly, and after living together for several weeks made a shocking revelation, "You know, Ellen," she began, "I used to be overweight." "Yeah, sure," Ellen replied, "Let me see now, you would consider yourself overweight if you cast a shadow, right?"

Rachel freely laughed at Ellen's dig. "No, really." Then looking into Ellen's eyes and deadly serious she said, "Ellen, I was bigger than you. There was a time when I tipped the scale at two hundred and fifty pounds," and with that she leaned forward and handed a photograph of herself to Ellen. "Please, never show this or mention this to anyone else."

Ellen could not catch the gasp before it escaped from her mouth. Here was her boney, little roommate Rachel in a costume of thick, misshapen flesh. "But how . . .," Ellen stammered.

Rachel then told her story, which paralleled Ellen's in many ways. Rachel had also been an overweight child and her parents had been mentally cruel as well as physically abusive. In the worst times of yelling and ridiculing, Rachel learned to keep eye contact with her mother or father while escaping to an inner world where she was the beautiful princess who had been kidnapped and raised by evil trolls. She fantasized her true father would find her, and then, empowered, she would have the trolls beheaded, be courted by a handsome prince, and live happily ever after.

As she got older, real life became more difficult and intrusive and the fantasies no longer worked. She realized that she would never be stronger than her parents or be able to change the ways that other people treated her. Then it occurred to her that the one thing she could change was herself. So every day she began to tell herself that the real evil in her life was food, especially sweets and fatty foods. Whenever she felt hunger pains, over and over in her mind she would repeat the phrase, "I hate food. It smells sick. It's full of nasty and disgusting refuse."

"The more I did this," Rachel said, "the more easily I was able to avoid food and pretty soon I began to lose weight." Even though Rachel's body was changing, her parents did not change—that is, they did not stop abusing her, they merely moved on to other things besides her weight. She no longer cared about what they said, because for the first time in her life she experienced something she had never known: hope, the kind of hope that springs from a sense of having control. She no longer felt powerless and all of this was new to her. Another first for her was the fact that she began to be noticed by boys.

Ellen was hooked. With Rachel's support and encouragement she could finally emerge from the darkness of her inner torment and self-loathing. Rather than hate herself, she would control herself. So she set out on a program of self-improvement through mind over meals, will over weight, and commitment over compromise.

What Rachel did not tell Ellen though, and did not yet fully realize, is that she had gone too far in her regimen and became anorexic. In fact, connective tissue in her joints had already begun to break down, her bones were becoming fragile, and her liver and kidneys were in the first stages of organ failure. What began for Rachel as self-improvement had become a form of self-destruction. Because of her irrational fear of ever again being even one ounce overweight, no one and nothing—not even her own physical demise—could persuade her to end her war on food.

Meanwhile, Ellen found the path of anorexia too difficult to travel. At first she was excited when she dropped a few pounds, but then her hunger became too great for her to ignore. She tried diet pills for awhile, but found that they made her feel too jittery and a couple of times she found herself out of breath and her heart racing without doing any sort of exercise. She was about to throw in the towel once again when she got her next big lesson in eating disorders (ED).

One day in the laundry room, one of the flighty students from the film school pulled Ellen's underwear out of her washer by mistake. "Whoa! These sure aren't mine. Who's got the hippo hidden in their room?" Then she looked at Ellen, and without any apology she said, "Here, these must be yours." Ellen was on the verge of hatred and a slow, torturous murder fantasy, but was immediately steered in a different direction when the girl continued, "I guess you haven't discovered the miracle of laxatives."

"What?" Ellen asked.

"Look, Chubby," the girl replied, "It's simple math. Your body turns calories into fat. No calories means no fat. So you eat as much as you want, eat until your sides ache, then you take enough laxatives to relieve a horse, and you don't gain an ounce. In fact, you lose weight."

Ellen wondered why she had never considered this equation before. "Yeah, I guess that makes sense."

"Of course it does. Some girls prefer to barf, but that's just too sick. It just takes a quick trip to the toilet and my weight is under control."

Ellen began her new campaign of body control, and within a few months boys were noticing her and if she did not still have such a poor self-image, she probably would have accepted a couple of dates. Every time she looked in the mirror though she still saw some place on her body where her fat continued to resist her attempt to starve it out—around her ankles, her inner thighs, the upper part of her arm that still wiggled when she lifted her hands over her head. The truth, however, is that Ellen had already dropped well below what would be considered a normal healthy weight, but her mind would not let her eyes see what everyone else saw when they looked at her. Failing to achieve body control through anorexia, Ellen found it in another, and equally destructive eating disorder, bulimia.

THE ONE-WAY TICKET DISORDER

Ellen, Rachel and the other coeds are composites of countless patients I have seen over the last couple of decades. These women, whose bodies and minds have been emaciated by ED's (eating disorders), have rarely come to my office by their own choice, but were dragged in by concerned parents, spouses, or their adult children. Some of them came in wheelchairs and others I saw for the first time were barely able to raise their heads from their hospital beds. Some did not receive professional help until it was too late and others died resisting treatment. ED's pose among the saddest and deadliest disorders that health professionals face today, and they are on the rise.

Tragically, serious illness and death are not uncommon consequences of ED, and the frustration for doctors is that we are often forced to stand by and helplessly watch people destroy themselves when we have much to offer in the way of healing. However, as most specialists can tell you, ED is among the most difficult disorders to treat, if not the most difficult, and it has one of the lowest success rates. In other words, once a woman (less frequently, a man) steps into the confused and complicated world of ED, the odds of spiraling downward are high. Seeking treatment, however, lessens this risk.

The general characteristics of an ED are:

- An abnormal preoccupation with weight and nutritional issues, which leads to other unhealthy behaviors.

- Obsessive thinking about body image and food are compounded when the diet is restricted.

- Obsessive thinking about body image and food are compounded with accompanying weight decrease (or, in some cases, increase).

- Obsessive thinking about body image and food are compounded by a cycle of binging and purging that becomes impossible to break.

Some women think losing a little weight will make them happy and become frustrated when they achieve this goal, but find they are no happier than before. They may decide at this point that they are on the right track, but they simply did not lose enough weight. However, once a person starts down that road, no amount of weight loss is ever enough. Does this sound unbelievable? I can tell you from experience that a young woman who, to you and I, looks like a living skeleton looks in a mirror and sees "just a few more places" on her body where she needs to lose "a little more fat." Once the ED reaches this level, the person's thinking becomes more clouded and distorted, and also becomes more difficult to treat. The patients who are the most treatment-resistant are those who have the longest histories of ED.

ED's are more complicated than any other disorder covered in this book, and that is why I have saved them for the second to the last chapter. They are not only the most complicated disorders to diagnose, but also the most difficult chemical imbalances to correct. In fact, ED's are more difficult to resolve than it is to break a drug addiction. The interplay between mind and body is especially intense in ED's, because in many cases the patients' minds literally make their eyes see distorted images of their bodies.

I suppose that by now you know me well enough to appreciate the fact that the inner-working of these patients' minds would naturally intrigue me and fuel my motivation to learn all I could about them. I am not only fascinated by the complexity of the spell these girls and women are under, but I have come to love them in the vulnerable and broken state that they sometimes do not even realize defines their lives.

In spite of the inherent frustrations that comes with treating every single patient with ED, the joy of making a positive difference in their mental, physical, relational, and spiritual health gives me the greatest satisfaction a human being could ever know.

WHO'S AT RISK?

An ED may begin as simply as the attempt to shed a couple of pounds to prepare for summer, a prom, or to improve ones performance in a time trial. While one girl will lose a pound and put it right back on, another will lose a pound and keep it off, and a third will lose a pound and begin to obsess over keeping that pound off and losing more weight. The girl who obsesses has taken her first step down the road of ED, from which she will not return without a great deal of pain, illness, grief, and damaged relationships. Of course, her chances of plunging from mere weight loss into a full-on ED is much greater if she already has an underlying mood disorder of some type.

ED's are far more common in females than in males, although I have had several male patients who have also suffered with this condition. Women generally are at highest risk sometime around adolescence, the onset being as early as prepubescent girls—eighty-one percent of ten-year-old girls are afraid of being fat—with the majority being several years after the onset of menses. ED's are not uncommon in adult women, many of whom continue to struggle with a persistent eating disorder (we may assume these women did not receive adequate treatment in the early stages of the disorder or became resistant to treatment early on). However, there are no healthy adult women with ED, because the nature of the disorder is both mentally and physically damaging. An ED is a killer.

SPORTS

Certain sports contribute a higher risk to the development of an eating disorder and a woman, or sometimes a man, who devote themselves to any sport, even jogging, runs the risk of suffering the consequences of ED. In 1994, Olympic gymnastic hopeful, Christy Henrich, died from an ED. She weighed sixty pounds. In 1997, Heidi Guenther, a ballerina from the Boston Ballet died at twenty-two years old from an ED. Other female deaths have been reported from not only gymnastics and dance, but also diving, track and field—any sport that requires maximum performance or a certain body-type for graceful appearance and movements. Boys and men can have eating disorder thinking and behaviors (though less likely) in these same sports, and also wrestling. Coaches, parents, judges, and peers are frequently responsible for pressuring athletes to lighter weights either to compete in lower divisions, to increase speed or agility, or to succeed at all costs.

Occasionally, the onset of an athlete's ED will follow an injury while recuperating, and exercise is out of the question. After working hard to develop lean muscle to excel in their sport, athletes hate to allow their bodies to put on fat, so sometimes they will rigorously restrict their food intake to compensate for their lack of exercise. When the body is healing itself, it needs extra resources and there is not much danger for a true athlete to take a hiatus long enough to fully heal, rehabilitate with physical therapy, and then return to training. Depending on the nature of the injury, all of this can occur within weeks to months. However, if an athlete eats significantly less food and is not smart about what kind of food is consumed, the subsequent weight loss may blind her to the fact that her injury did not heal as well as it should have and she has begun to suffer from malnutrition, which had interfered greatly with the normal healing process.

Many people who either want to live healthier lives or lose weight begin programs every month of monitoring their diets and regular exercise. For most people—who continue with these programs until they become habitual—they achieve their goals without any negative consequences. However, there are those others who cross the line that separates healthy from unhealthy behavior. Their diet becomes too severe and their exercise becomes too frenetic until they end up destroying and deforming their bodies rather than healing and beautifying them. The tragedy is that by the time they get to this point, their brain is so deprived of nutrients, and it has been trapped in a warped mind-set for so long, they cannot see how damaged they have become.

MEDIA

Thumb through a teen magazine sometime and look at the advertisements. What messages and stories are being told in the photographs? What messages are being communicated to eleven-, twelve-, and thirteen-year-old girls? Basically, the media tells them over and over again, that image is their identity and if they want to be liked, they had better be thin. What benefit is it to teenage girls (and their younger sisters), or to society, if they are given the impression that they are unattractive if their bodies carry an ounce of extra weight? What is there to be gained from a girl being terrified that she will not be accepted by her peers for having the wrong type of body?

Of course, advertisers prey on the fears of us all. By creating self-doubts and insecurities about our social status, leveraging our emotional uncertainties against images of popularity, and offering promises of fulfilling relationships or fairytale romances, marketers exploit the psychological needs of adolescents on behalf of their clients. In doing so, they not only create consumers for products, they also create illusions that young people mistake for reality. Attempting to conform to that reality leads to self-destruction.

The modeling industry is, of course, notorious for perpetuating ED's and there are woeful tales of models who eat diet pills like candy and faint on sets for lack of energy from not eating. As long as these gaunt images are held up as the symbols of beauty, garbed in the latest fashions by the world's best designers, young women are going to hear society's message loud and clear, regardless of what we tell them. One cannot help but wonder when someone is going to poll the average American Joe as to what he thinks about a little extra flesh, roundness, softness, and shapely body contour, as opposed to boney bodies and skull-like heads.

Family and Childhood Environments

The family frequently contributes a great deal to the patient's ED, especially if there is a history of mood disorders. However, aside from chemical imbalances, a family's psychological and relational dynamics can undermine a child's self-esteem, leaving her vulnerable to an ED in order to cope with feelings of inadequacy.

For example, many dads and brothers are clueless as to when their teasing has gone over the line and becomes torture. What was "just having some fun" for them was taken seriously and literally by the daughter or sister. A negative comment about the girl's weight, while pinching her side or slapping her butt, can be interpreted in her mind as the way she is seen by all men. In fact, a daughter's relationship with her father is her first and primary exposure, not only to men and the way they think, but also to the way she appears in the eyes of men. To the father who adores his daughter and accepts her unconditionally, a young woman generally has a healthy sense of who she is apart from her body image. However, a father who makes a girl's body image an issue has already set her up for future heartaches and problems and a lifetime of striving to be "good enough."

Whatever nurturing and positive attention a girl, and later the young woman, does not receive from her father, she will likely look for it from other boys and men. Unfortunately, she will often seek to win the favor of the very same type of man her father is. For example, if her father's personality is distant or mean, she will be drawn to a man with the same disposition. Because they are starved for attention, do not feel good about themselves, and may not want to be alone, they can be easy prey for those men who are controlling. One abusive relationship can tend to lead to another, and disappointment is added to disappointment, until the young woman feels her life has slipped completely out of her control and is completely worthless.

The mother's role is also crucial as the primary caretaker of the daughter. Again, there are mothers who do an excellent job of instilling confidence and self-esteem in their daughters, encouraging them to develop the life of the mind and soul and not merely the shape of the body. There are also moms who make thoughtless comments like, "You are never going to get a boyfriend looking like that!" or "Why don't you try to drop a few pounds, sweetheart, so maybe some-one will ask you out."

ED patients may be trying to please parents who are not easily pleased and, no matter what they do, it is never enough. Other patients have been sexually abused by a family member, and, like other ED cases, they use their disorder as a means of control. Unable to exercise control over what is going on outside, around, or even to them, they control the one thing they found they can control, their weight.

We all have a psychological need to feel that we are in control of something. Some people have a greater need to feel that they are in control than others. These people also feel the need to control a greater number of events, objects, and relationships in their lives—they are looking to micro-control their world. Most of us live with an acceptable compromise between the things we control and resignation over the things we cannot control. However, a human life without any control is unthinkable. The opposite of control is not simply powerlessness, but also hopelessness and despair.

One of the doctor's responsibilities with ED patients is to let them know it is our job to help them get control of their lives. We need to let them know that we require their help in this process. Since we are working on their lives, it is crucial that they are ultimately in control. We are simply there to help them put their lives back into their own hands. As best we can, we need to enlighten them to the fact that they are being controlled by the disorder and we will help them put an end to that ruthless regime. Some patients become very disturbed when they realize they were not in control as much as they had assumed. On the other hand, for those who begin to get the vision of being in control of their lives—rather than just their bodies—for the first time experience the hope they need for the difficult battle that lies ahead.

Everything we say to them should serve to inspire hope. For this reason we can encourage these patients that the process of recovery is doable if, with all their heart, they will apply themselves to the treatment. Assuring them that this challenge is like other difficult tasks they have already accomplished in their lives, we empower them to take the upper hand over this disorder. This kind of pep talk is especially effective with patients who are perfectionists and enjoy taking on a good challenge.

If an ED patient is someone who was physically, emotionally, verbally, or sexually abused during her childhood, and control over her body and actions were denied her, then she may have grabbed on to her ED as a means of taking over something she could control—what goes in and what comes out. This may sound bizarre, and indeed it is, but it is not uncommon for ED patients to pay careful attention not only to what they eat, but also to their purging (such as vomiting) and bowel movements and so on. Because many of them use excessive amounts of laxatives or binge on junk foods, it is not uncommon for them to experience frequent diarrhea and constipation, with bloating and pain. They tend to have more than an average awareness, and control over, what goes into their bodies and how it goes out. This gives them a sense of power.

Peer pressure plays a major role, especially in preadolescence—the sixth to eighth grades—as students become self-conscious and begin to compare themselves to others. Sadly, their emotional perspective often clouds and overshadows their reason, so that they are not able to make accurate assessments about themselves and what attributes or characteristics they can boast in their favor. If they have an outstanding talent in athletics, academics, or they are attractive, or their peers are kind—certainly a rarity on most junior high school campuses—then they may have a chance to find their own arena in which to shine. Otherwise, they are likely to hear again and again, in one way or another, that they are an outsider, inadequate, unattractive, and unwanted.

Something Quite Unexpected

Believe it or not, a girl (or boy) can begin to obsess over food simply from what she learns or experiences in a nutrition class at school. While most students would find a class on healthy eating helpful and informative, some young women (or young men) can become alarmed by side remarks the teacher may make regarding weight gain, skin complexion, or cancer. The student then begins to carefully read the labels on every jar, can, and package of any food item before she decides whether she will eat it or not. Given the state of today's processed foods, additives, preservatives, and inclusions of more glucose and sodium than most humans need, her range of acceptable intake narrows more and more. Some patients go "vegan" or more extreme forms of vegetarianism, while in actuality a well-balanced diet works the best and is the healthiest and most healthy way to live. However, because she is not well informed on her body's need for protein and amino acids, essential minerals, as well as the good fats and cholesterols, she is unaware of how she is depriving her body of the necessary food sources for maintaining bone and tissue strength as well as organ function. In this case, a class that was intended to promote nutrition and health turned out to be her introduction to ED.

When these disorders go untreated early on, the chance that they will persist and become more severe increases every year, sometimes exponentially. The more time that passes, and the more ingrained the behavior becomes, the more difficult it is to treat. Early treatment is not simply a matter of better education and nutrition, but correcting a distortion in the patient's thinking, and the earlier this happens the better the prognosis for a total recovery. Still, even recovered patients admit that ED lingers as a problem that frequently enters their minds.

Although it would be a mistake to make hard, fast rules from generalizations, the majority of ED patients come from families with incomes in the upper percentile. The patients themselves are likely to be high achievers academically, intelligent, and feel pressured to live up to unrealistic expectations that they have set for themselves or perceive that others have set for them. Unfortunately their perceptions are sometimes correct, in that their parents, teachers, or coaches make mental or physical demands on them that push them beyond their normal limits. If these conditions coincide with low self-esteem, the child is more likely to succumb to an ED than if she has a positive self-image and is self-confident. Also, the greater her own desire or feeling of responsibility to please her parents, the greater her liability to snap. ED's are the disorder of choice for young women who struggle emotionally, physically, relationally, socially, and spiritually.

Going Too Far

So far I have generalized ED's, but have mostly had anorexia in mind. The literal meaning of anorexia is "without appetite," but that is misleading in light of what women who suffer from this condition are doing to themselves. We could more accurately define anorexia as a form of self-starvation, usually due to an irrational fear of being overweight. Initially the anorexic may find herself constantly famished, but there are strange symptoms brought on by this condition that alter the patient's attitude toward food, others and herself.

Some anorexics come to a point where they hate food and can barely tolerate the smell of it or can eat it only when it is specially prepared. Others experience a kind of euphoria or spaced-out feeling that results from depriving their brains of the nutrients necessary to think clearly. There are patients who appreciate this by-product of anorexia, because it creates in them a sense of distance from their own emotions. However, that is not to say mood disorders are less severe in anorexic patients, because just the opposite can be true. Rather, the scope of their emotions is not as broad and therefore appears more manageable, and control and manageability is exactly what many of these women are attempting to achieve.

If not for the irrational thinking that is associated with ED, no one could possibly believe that self-starvation is a cure for any sort of personal problem. We do not have our arms amputated because our hand itches, so why starve and destroy our entire body because our hearts ache, a few of our relationships aren't working, or we do not look like the emaciated models who pose in magazines? We are wiser, instead, to deal with the underlying problems, with the first order of business being to correct chemical imbalances that prevent us from seeing clearly and making the best possible decisions.

Anorexics can be extremely difficult patients to treat, because they did not master the battle of self-starvation by being weak-willed. Even if they smile and act pleasant in the office, the anorexic has already made up her (unstable) mind that she is going to continue to avoid eating. If she is able to do this through hunger pains and her physical drive and need for self-preservation, then she will often be more than a match for the doctor in the relatively short amount of time they have together.

The Food Fix

In the complex inner world of our nervous system, the balance of conditions critical to life—such as body temperature, blood flow to organs, heart rate, and so on—is maintained by the tension of two opposing forces. Think of it like this: You are going to take a shower, so you turn on the hot water faucet. After awhile though the water temperature is too hot, so you turn on the cold water faucet. Soon the water is too cool, so you adjust the hot water. You continue to test the water temperature, make adjustments to both valves, and in a moment or two you have the exact temperature you desire.

The brain performs these types of monitoring and adjusting functions for your body twenty-four hours a day your entire life, constantly making minute adjustments to maintain a stable balance (referred to as homeostasis). Instead of using hot and cold, the brain has a remarkable chemistry set that interacts with various functions of the body. Some chemicals serve to turn on a system (for example, release white blood cells to fight an infection) while others serve to turn off a system. The tension between the chemicals that work against each other, so to speak, in turning on and turning off a system is what keeps those systems balanced-like keeping the water in the shower the perfect temperature.

Sometimes the body experiences a sudden fright that calls for an immediate response. For example, drivers may need to slam on their brakes to avoid a serious collision. When this happens, the brain releases a chemical (catecholamine, better known as adrenaline) into the central nervous system to produce the necessary response. Immediately the entire body is on high energy alert. Not knowing what will come next, but recognizing imminent danger, the body prepares to mobilize and burn fuel as quickly as possible. Also, the brain will ask the body to ingest the kind of food that can be quickly metabolized and turned into useful energy (coincidentally, this is also the same type of food that is most easily stored as fat). The body undergoes other dramatic and sudden changes that we do not notice until the threat has passed—for example, the adrenaline rush, racing heart, and rapid breathing, all produced by a chemical triggering device.

Once the "event" has passed, the body has to recover its normal state, otherwise to remain in heightened readiness would eventually begin to wear it down. Another chemical is then released by the brain to counteract the earlier chemical and return the nervous system to its normal state of rest and digest.

What happens to a nervous system if it is placed in a situation in which it is constantly or frequently receiving the signal to prepare for quick action? This would include such situations as a demanding job that we hate, having a boss or supervisor who is an oppressive jerk, parents who are abusive, and the many other conditions that we have come to accept as normal life in the twenty-first century. What happens is that the nervous system is always hyped up without sufficient counter-balancing mechanisms to bring it down. Or, in the analogy of the shower, the hot tap is always open and the cold tap is either shut off, slightly open, or open and closed intermittently, but not enough to ever produce the perfect temperature.

Our brain knows when our body is out of balance. Our brain also knows that it is responsible to do something about the imbalance. In order to resolve the nervous system's high demand for fuel foods, the body goes looking for carbohydrates, and for most of us it does not have to look very far before it finds a bag of chips, a jar of cookies, a quart of ice cream, or a cheap hamburger. These are exactly the foods the brain needs to produce endorphins (a biochemical that naturally produces feelings of relief and pleasure) and affect levels of serotonin, dopamine and the other chemicals. In other words, the high-carbohydrate fuels that the nervous system craves are comfort foods or *stress eating*, because they assist the brain in counteracting the effects of ongoing stress. They also serve to provide a lonely or unhappy person with a moment of pleasure in a world of misery.

Of course, foods that add excess weight (fat) to our bodies, and run the risk of cardiovascular disease or stroke, are not the only solutions to the problem. Even moderate exercise, like a walk around the block, is a much healthier way to produce endorphins. So are relaxation exercises, a massage, sitting in a hot tub, and sex. The point is, many people use food to counteract feelings of unrelenting stress, unhappiness, or boredom when food is a short-term "fix" and not a cure.

The ED patients who overeat and tend to eat foods that are stored as fat rather than useful to their body's needs are generally overweight—unless they are using a method of purging to prevent weight gain. As they put on the pounds, their level of activity decreases. They find that walking up a flight of stairs has them out of breath and any exercise that is more strenuous is bound to result in fatigue and pain. Some may attempt an exercise routine, but generally, on close review, it tends to be too insufficient to compensate for their food intake.

The reason some of these patients cannot break free (and it is not an exaggeration to compare their condition to an addiction in respect to their physical and mental cravings), is because hidden among all the other factors contributing to their ED is a mood disorder. I hope that some day everyone has a much better education in how important a healthy diet is to brain function and how some mental conditions can be resolved with a proper balance of vitamins, minerals and proteins. EDs are notorious for causing confusion, poor judgment, irrational thinking, and other conditions that interfere with normal brain functions. Therefore, it is not surprising that ED patients sometimes think they are hungry when in truth they are sad or depressed. Therefore, they are turning to food when they should be turning to something that will help to promote a real cure.

When I introduce ED patients to mood normalizing medications, I explain to them that I am not offering them "crutches." They need to understand that their emotional eating has been a form of self-medication that has not worked, does not work, and will never work. However, when together we have brought their neurochemicals into a proper balance, their metabolism will improve, they will have more energy, their appetite will decrease (or increase if appropriate), and their motivation will increase. Getting the chemical part of their condition resolved will go a long way in bringing them to the place where they will be able to tackle the physical part of their health care on their own.

THE OSCILLATORS

There are ED patients who, unlike anorexics, do not starve themselves, and unlike bulimics, binge, but do not gain weight. First, there are the "yo-yo" dieters who put themselves on strict diets—either following the latest trend or inventing their own "plan"—and after they have made a little progress they decide they can cheat on their diet "just a little," or it is time to reward themselves, or they are simply too hungry and weak to deny themselves any longer. Then they feast like an emperor at a Roman banquet. Since they feel like they have been really good for long enough, they feel justified in eating excessive amounts of sugars and other unhealthy foods. After awhile though, they begin to feel sluggish, their clothes are tight again, and guilt returns. Now they are back at the beginning of the cycle, preparing themselves for another lap in a race that will take them nowhere and for which they will eventually pay in the loss of quality of life, health, and possibly an early death.

The behavior of a second type of oscillator sounds bizarre when you first hear of it, but is very common: bulimia nervosa. If you imagine watching the first type of oscillator in fast or in time-lapse photography, you have an idea of bulimia, because what the first type might do over months, the bulimic will do in twenty-four hours without dieting and with or without exercise. Bulimia is characterized by binge eating followed by purging—that is, emptying the contents of the stomach either by the use of laxatives, by inducing vomiting or by over-exercising, or in whichever way the individual's neurochemical imbalances present both emotionally and physically. There are women with bulimia who binge and purge several times a day. Some who experience increased weight gain may become desperate and increase the behaviors that don't work and that cause the same recurring problems, creating a vicious cycle that is hard to break and others who take up to a hundred laxatives a day, while keeping an exercise regimen of two to three or more hours every day. Some bulimics eat an enormous amount of food knowing they will get rid of it as soon as they have finished their meal. In their minds, they have "the best of both worlds": they get to gorge themselves on foods they enjoy and then they get to enjoy the relief—and for some, "pleasure"—of getting rid of it.

Bulimic patients can become so obsessive that they will purge even small amounts of food eaten during the day, reducing their caloric intake to a dangerously low level. Although all bulimics put themselves at high risk for serious medical problems (more and more insurance companies are backing away from covering EDs), the younger patients are amazingly resilient. Young and otherwise healthy bodies may be able to handle the abuse inflicted on them before the grim results appear. However, they are usually oblivious to the permanent damage they are doing to themselves and, sadly, I have seen several deaths resulting from the unhealthy behaviors associated with bulimia.

Paradoxically, like the food fix patients, bulimics can also find comfort in purging and use it as a means of temporarily easing stress, while others purge out of feelings of boredom or loneliness. In the same way that the brain can adapt to the oversupply of chemicals provided by comfort foods, binging and purging can produce an immediate yet brief feeling of pleasure, which some patients describe as a "high." Like other addictive behaviors, the brain can build tolerance to this high, requiring more frequent episodes to achieve the same results, until the pleasure is replaced by a compulsive habit.

Some bulimic patients struggle with their disorder because they believe it to be not only unhealthy, but morally wrong. Therefore, they will resist purging, promise themselves they will never do it again, but at some point break down and find themselves guilt-ridden at the beginning of another cycle of self-loathing, desperate resistance and a build up of stress and pressure, which leads to another episode of giving in to the disorder. Other bulimics find relief in punishing themselves by inducing vomiting, since they feel guilty about eating too much. Evacuating the excessive amount of food they have eaten provides relief from guilt by giving them a sense of undoing their wrong (or sinful) behavior. However, in the next moment guilt returns because they now feel bad about the purging, and they take that next step in the big circle in which they are forever running.

Most ED patients do not even know that they have gone too far with their weight loss until after enduring months of being pestered by their friends and family with annoying questions, like "How much longer are you supposed to be on this ridiculous diet?" "Do you feel alright?" and "Don't you think it's time to see a doctor?" Even then, the patient shakes her head, unable to comprehend why all the fuss and why everyone has to be so unreasonable. She looks in the mirror and sees a body that needs trimming and severe discipline to be kept under control, while everyone else seems to think she looks ill. Like everyone else with an ED, her condition is integrally bound up with her body and her sense of self-esteem.

Women with ED's are generally affected by a condition known to doctors as body dysmorphism: the form of their body appears to them as an exaggeration of how it actually looks. When they look in the mirror, they do not see themselves dangerously—and unattractively—underweight, yet that is how they appear to the rest of the world. Their mind has not only warped their body image, but they have lost touch with reality to such a degree that the opinion and consensus of other people is likely to make little difference to their way of thinking. Quite often, neither a loving family member nor an objective professional physician can get through to them. She may continue to point to a part of her body and say, "See this? This is simply too fat." In focusing on that one area though, she loses sight of the rest of her body to the detriment of the whole.

SIGNS AND SYMPTOMS

There are more subtle forms of ED that a doctor or family member can easily overlook or dismiss as "not serious enough to worry about," yet still threatens the patient's quality of life. In fact, the majority of ED patients' behavior can be easily hidden. For example, anorexic patients may be only ten to twenty pounds under their ideal body weight and those with bulimia may be normal weight, underweight, or even slightly overweight (purging once or twice a week or less as opposed to those who purge several times a day). We have to be alert to the subtle signs of ED's. This is especially important for doctors since the time they have to spend with their patients is sometimes too brief.

One common characteristic of ED patients is that they will resist being weighed during an office visit. Sometimes the office staff will allow a patient to waive off stepping on the scale, saying something like, "My weight never changes. It's exactly the same as my last visit. Don't make me step on that stupid thing again." In this situation, our suspicion is not aroused by a change in weight so much as the patient's unwillingness to have this aspect of her health measured or to have her weight known to anyone else.

Another characteristic is that ED patients will often obsess over their weight, constantly counting calories and investigating the latest diets. Even if thin (or too thin) already, they will ask the doctor if there are any new medications that will help them boost their metabolism and burn more fat. When a young woman who is not overweight asks these types of questions, doctors need to begin asking "innocent" questions that will indicate whether addressing an ED might be appropriate.

Of course, patients who are significantly underweight, but are not aware of being below average or do not agree with the doctor that they are, should be prime suspects. The same is true of patients who demonstrate sudden or dramatic weight loss. Also, such things as skin and muscle tone are affected by deprivation of necessary nutrients, so the physical presentation of the patient can be another indicator. Serious ED's will also have damaging effects on the patients' teeth and bulimics, in particular, frequently suffer severe tooth decay from vomiting.

Suspicion should be raised by patients who substitute coffee or other caffeinated and high energy drinks for regular meals. Then there are those ED patients who isolate themselves, living lonely and depressed lives, longing to be accepted by others, but are too fearful of rejection to venture out into public. Because these women allow themselves to be defined by body image, it is not unusual for them to feel worthless and show symptoms of low self-esteem.

Physically, they will sometimes present with migraine headaches, confusion, or dizziness. They may suffer stomach cramps, heart irregularities, a body temperature that is below average, or broken blood vessels in their eyes due to frequent purging. In many cases, their immune systems have been severely compromised for lack of nutrition required to keep it in peak condition. Another rather serious symptom appears when a woman does not ingest an adequate supply of healthy fats and protein, and this is especially true of female athletes who tend to burn off everything they eat. Without a healthy percentage of body fat, the female body is unable to produce normal amounts of estrogen, and may miss periods or even stop menstruating. The longer a young woman goes without a period, the more serious the damaging consequences are likely to be later on. ED patients tend to fear that the fat they eat will make them "fat." It is important, however, to recognize this is not true.

Some patients may develop parotid gland swelling which can cause their faces to swell. Swelling can also occur in other areas of their bodies due to fluid retention. Generally, they are not at all happy with their physical appearance when this happens, because it looks to them like they are getting "fat." Unfortunately, this mistaken assumption drives them to more drastic food restrictions or more frequent purging, which will, of course, fail to resolve the problem, but instead just makes it worse.

One of the complications of ED's is that their emotional symptoms can mimic mood disorders, such as anxiety, irritability, and depression, while other patients show no indication of an underlying mood disorder. Diagnosis is even more difficult with patients whose changes in weight or behavior occur gradually over time. However, a doctor or family member who is alert to the symptoms above will, hopefully, have the advantage of detecting it early, which makes all the difference in both recovery of health and the success of treatment for eating disorders.

As I said before, an ED is a killer. Imagine a disease that causes the deterioration of every organ in the body, that weakens bones, and deprives the skin all that it needs to stay supple and resist infection. Anyone in her right mind who was diagnosed with this disease would want to seek help. But "right mind" becomes one of the casualties of the ED. The ED patient needs to know and understand the damage she is doing to herself and that she is committing suicide, but in a very slow fashion.

Some patients are motivated to slow down or curtail their ED once they have been educated to its consequences. Being momentarily scared though does not always prove to result in long-term changes, and ED's in every respect, including treatment, are a long-term consideration. Once the fear wears off, the greater pressures of wanting to look a particular way and not seeing their desired form in their reflection causes them to return to their self-destructive pattern. However, if terrifying them with the truth can serve as a motivator to awaken them from their stupor and get them started on the road to recovery, I advocate being truthful and honest even if they find it upsetting. For some patients, it will just take that first step in the right direction, and then the momentum of healing will take over.

The Consequences of ED: Firm But Fair

There are many things about ED that patients do not know, but need to learn. If it helps to get their attention long enough to consider getting help, then a crash course of the consequences of their actions is in order. For example, most women with bulimia do not know that they will put on more fat weight over time. When I present this information to patients, they find it difficult to believe and some have thought I was trying to pull some trick on them. The truth is, though, that when the body is being starved it will do all it can to store fat since it does not know when it will be fed again. In fact, the body will rob muscles of protein to burn for energy rather than utilize fat cells, saving fat for emergencies.

Secondly, the organs of the body must be nourished to function. If they are starved, they will begin to shut down to conserve energy. If an organ's function drops low enough it may be difficult to bring it back up again. Because the kidneys and liver are not functioning at healthy levels, the ED patients are likely to retain more fluid (and toxins) the longer they continue with this behavior. They are also likely to experience decreased bowel motility, which causes bloating and other symptoms that lead to an increase in weight and an unsightly body image. The idea of putting on weight and losing control over their body's metabolism may be unacceptable, and they may try to avoid this at all costs. The body does not know what to do next if it has received too many mixed signals.

I usually explain how bowel dysfunction causes an imbalance in electrolytes, such as sodium, potassium and others, which in turn adversely affects the body's fluids and tissues. Bowel function becomes more irregular and can cause alternating bouts of constipation and diarrhea. Bowel dysfunction intensifies their symptoms and results in abdominal pain, gas, bloating, acid reflux, hemorrhoids, bleeding, and other symptoms related to irritation of the bowels. Some patients try to correct these problems with laxatives, but do even more damage to their bodies, because helping the bowels in this way reduces their ability to function properly on their own. This unhealthy behavior related to ED confuses the body and disrupts its natural metabolism. The idea of putting on weight and losing control over their bodies through the very mechanisms they have used to get control is enough to convince some patients to pay attention since that is exactly what the patient fears and wants to avoid.

Many ED patients have to curtail and limit exercise to levels that their bodies can tolerate. Because of the weakened condition of their bones and muscles due to malnutrition, any extra stress through over-exercise places them at a higher risk for fractures from falls, compression fractures of the spine, and other complications. They need to understand that they are compromising their chances of participating in sports in both the near and distant future if their condition is not corrected. Again, there are some patients for whom athletic activity is so important, that they will take this information very seriously and be more likely to cooperate with a treatment program.

ED patients are at high risk for bone disease and generally experience a thinning of bone density (osteopenia and osteoporosis). Young women with osteoporosis may receive the same treatment as elderly women who, by reason of age, have lower hormone levels and therefore require supplements and agents that are effective in strengthening bones. However, a normal, healthy young woman should never have to consider such things if she is on a balanced diet. Patients who develop osteoporosis relatively early in life can limit their body's ability to grow to its full potential height. If these patients could hear the others who suffer with osteoporosis talk about how they wish they had known the permanent harm they were doing to their bodies, they would have made changes long ago. We are doing our patients a great favor in warning them ahead of time. However, reason does not go far, unfortunately, in winning over an irrational mind.

Eating disorders must be treated aggressively, but, at the same time, we must not push these patients so hard that we scare them off. When talking over their ED with them, my goal is to be firm but fair, to cover the critical issues of their disorder, but listen to the pain or despair that has driven them to this behavior in the first place. If I listen well to what they have to say, I can respond sympathetically and offer them an alternative to dealing with their problems that does not include decimating their bodies.

Many women with ED have probably never stopped to think about the long-term and internal consequences of their actions. Once the obsessive behavior takes over, their thinking patterns become controlled by the disorder, because they constantly have to hide it, explain (lie about) it, and maintain it. In this regard, the behavior of an ED is similar to the habit of smoking: it is easier to start than to stop, and even if they quit for awhile, there is a great temptation to revert to those old habits during times of stress. For this reason, we must make every effort to stop the thinking patterns and behaviors early on, because the longer they persist, the more difficult they are to change.

"The Pill" (And Why It Can Help)

As with every other aspect of treating patients with mood and eating disorders, the doctor's medical service to the patient includes education. This is especially true when I prescribe an oral contraceptive along with mood normalizing medications. This may only be necessary if there is an absence of menses or if her cycles are irregular. Some patients' faces go pale when I mention the pill, and parents have become irate before hearing my reasoning. Typical responses and concerns to prescribing the pill to young women with ED include:

- The pill is against our religion.
- Won't I gain weight if I'm on the pill?
- Are you implying that our daughter is sexually active?
- We're afraid that if she is on the pill, she will become sexually active.

I am not in a position to debate religion, but most priests and ministers will make exceptions if they know that the pill is being used for medicinal purposes and not as a contraceptive, that it will be used only as long as necessary (which may not be more than two or three months), and if the patient's physical health and ongoing healing can be greatly enhanced by taking it. If this is a problem, first listen carefully to what the doctor has to say about using the pill, and then take that information to your spiritual teacher or counselor (or give that person this book with this chapter marked) and seek their advice.

The pill does not necessarily result in weight gain. That old complaint has been resolved with newer versions of the pill that have less hormones that could result in putting on extra weight. Doctors who know the patients' worries can work out a program and prescription that will alleviate the problem. If a woman is worried about water retention weight, she can make a point to drink more water and be careful in monitoring her salt intake.

Research among adolescents who take oral contraceptives for medical reasons has shown that they do not become any more sexually active than their peers. Besides, the unfortunate truth is that teenagers who become sexually active do not make that decision based on birth control, because they usually do not think that far in advance. That is one reason why there are so many teen pregnancies.

Whether a doctor, patient, parent, or minister, the biggest concern should be only for the young woman's health. With this in view, the pill may be an important addition to optimize the effectiveness of the overall treatment. If the patient still does not want to be on the pill, I let her know that as soon as her nutrition is balanced and her body fat is adequately increased I will then consider having her discontinue it and see whether it is still needed.

The truth is, birth control is not always a bad idea for some of these young women, because their low self-esteem and need for attention makes them more susceptible to coercion. A boyfriend, for example, may have much more influence on the patient's decision-making than any other person in her life. If a girl discovers that boys notice her when she dresses "sexy," she may attract someone whose only interest in her is using her for his own gratification. Craving attention and hating the idea of being alone or "the only girl without a boyfriend," she may not be able to come up with a good enough reason to turn down a young man's advances. Also, an adolescent boy who recognizes a girl's vulnerability and intends to exploit it, is likely to be sexually aggressive and unwilling to take "No" for an answer.

Since this is a sensitive issue, if I discern that the patient could face sexual risks if on the pill, I will have a private discussion with her. However, if she indicates that she and her parents are already conversing on this subject and is willing to have them in the room, then we will all engage in the discussion. Nevertheless, in most cases it is important to find opportunities to speak privately with these patients, assuring them of confidentially. They tend to have many thoughts that they keep to themselves, but, because their thinking is unhealthy, it is vital that they bring those issues to light and receive the counsel and insight of others. Open communication leads to better results, because the trust that the patients learn to place in the doctor increases the possibility they will follow the treatment plan. So, doctors must prove to them, in actions and not merely words, that we have their best interests in mind and our goal is to help them become as healthy as possible.

The "Why" of the Pill in Treating Eating Disorders

Quite simply, for underweight women who, due to malnutrition, are unable to menstruate on their own, hormonal replacement is a crucial move in supplying their bodies with what they need to function, recover, and return to a healthy state. This can be accomplished through oral contraceptives, which may have value for both short-term and long-term improvement.

One important reason for addressing hormone replacement is the patient's bone mass, especially in younger women still in a critical time of physical development. Increased levels of estrogen—i.e., bringing them up to the normal range—has the added benefit of improving the patient's mood, even as we have seen during estrogen therapy for postmenopausal women. Another benefit is restoring patterns of clearer thinking, which is invaluable when it comes to them making evaluations and decisions on their own, as all of us must do every day.

However, our goal is not to replace menses, but to recover it so that the patient returns to a normal cycle without an oral contraceptive. The way we go about restoring regular periods is through a strategic program of nutritional changes. The body must carry enough fat to convert into estrogen so that the body's needs are met and normal menses resumes. If when she has gained a sufficient level of body fat, but menses has still not resumed, I will have the patient discontinue the pill and wait to see if her periods will start again naturally. If it is ready, her body should tell itself to do so once it is no longer receiving hormones from the outside, although it may take a month or two. We may have to have several of these trial runs before we have achieved our goal, and the whole process can take months to a year or more. However, in resolving critical hormonal and endocrine problems, patience is a virtue that plays out well for the patient in the long run.

There is no need to rush to the pill. If a patient's condition indicates that she is close to resuming her period, the doctor may choose to postpone an oral contraceptive until it is known one way or another how to proceed. If a patient does not want to take the pill, then letting her know that if she can get her body to resume menses through eating right and following the rest of the doctor's instructions, she will not have to take the pill, which may provide added incentive for her to comply.

However, we cannot wait indefinitely for her period to return, because each month that passes can result in additional weakening of the bones. Sometimes it is helpful to conduct a body fat analysis to determine how close a patient may be to achieving menses, and it never hurts to consult a nutritionist for the best dietary advice. We may check a DEXA (bone density scan) diagnostically or as a baseline to follow later. There are exceptions to the rule, but most women can have periods if they have at least eighteen percent body fat—a few others may menstruate at a lower percentage. The minimum, however, is not optimum health, and a better low-range body fat percentage would be more like twenty to twenty-two percent. ED patients will, of course, want their fat percentage as low as possible and will make every effort to stay at the lower end of normal, or just below that. As a result, it is common, then, for them to have irregular menstrual cycles with some lapses lasting three or four months between menses.

Short-term vs Long-term Thinking

Recovery from an ED is extremely difficult in our instant gratification culture. The process is long and requires a great deal of ongoing dedication, self-discipline, and motivation. To have strong support from doctors, family and friends— which is not always the case—is invaluable to their progress. We cannot measure their recovery in months or years, because, like the addict or alcoholic, it is for the remainder of their lives.

Adolescents with an ED face an added challenge, making it even more difficult for them to fight their way to full remission than older women. We have discovered their unique situation, in part, from magnetic resonance imaging (MRI). The teenage brain is a work in progress, development beginning in the back of the brain to the front, and it is related to maturity. Why is this important? Because the frontal lobes of the human brain handle the executive functions, such as self-discipline, judgment, future planning, decision-making, impulse control, and delayed gratification. Adolescents are ill-equipped to voluntarily take on challenges that require long-range planning and working hard today for rewards that will not be enjoyed until months or years from now. The front part of the brain is usually not fully developed until people are in their mid-twenties. The maturity factor relating to delayed gratification helps to explain both the reason why so many young women fall prey to ED's and why it is so difficult for them to recover from them. We may add to this deficit the tragedy of what self-starvation does to the brain in diminishing its resources and functions.

We are not surprised that many adults with ED's exhibit an adolescent mindset and is, therefore, another argument for addressing these conditions as early as possible. Initially, self-starvation will halt the brain's development, so the patient gets stuck at that emotional maturity level (as is the case with all other addictions). As the condition continues, her mental functions will eventually regress and her reasoning and judging skills will deteriorate.

Doctors and parents can go a long way in helping an adolescent improve if we learn to speak in terms that young women can understand. For instance, I have explained to young women who hope to have babies later in life, that they could find it difficult to conceive if their menstrual imbalance, due to malnutrition, is not corrected. In fact, if they were going to ever get pregnant, their normal cycle would have to resume. Otherwise, conceiving a child is impossible. Of course there are young women who are not interested in having children or the thought of being "that old" seems remote—which is the same reason it is difficult to get adolescent smokers to give up cigarettes; if they get cancer or suffer heart disease or respiratory problems, it seems so far in the future as to be incomprehensible. For them, everything is short-term. If her future ability to conceive is not important to her at that time, I will try to figure out what is important to her—athletics, physical beauty, doing good for others, quality of life, critical thinking, and so on—and present to her the big picture of a whole life as opposed to the relatively small period of time of life of the preteen and teen years. Whatever can be used as a motivator, short of verbal or physical abuse, should be considered only because these patients can be so extremely difficult to reach.

Family Matters

If an adolescent patient is brought to the office by her parents, doctors can use their first visit as an opportunity to observe the family's interaction and gain information that will be helpful in moving forward with an effective program. In my practice, I will first greet the patient while making eye contact and then meet anyone else who is in the room. Next, I ask the patient to describe her problem or symptoms and tell me how I can help. The whole time I am observing how the patient responds, if she looks nervously away from me, looks to a parent as if pleading for help, or if they snap at me with an angry response. Some parents will ask the girl to do the talking, while others jump right in and talk for her. Patients who maintain eye contact with me, and are able to clearly explain why they are there, tells me something about their confidence and self-esteem.

Anger is not unusual, both in the patient's body language and speech. Sometimes the patient's anger is directed toward her parents, whom they have come to hate. Frequently they extend those negative feelings toward the doctor, who is seen either as an accomplice or, perhaps, the source of all the problems. Friction between the parents and patients can be very uncomfortable, but it is also a lesson the doctor is learning that will help unlock the best approach to treating the ED. Some young women have directed all of their hostility towards me, and are the angriest as well as the most difficult to treat.

A good gauge to determine how deep these patients are into their ED and if they are already motivated to get better is to ask them, "Do you feel that you have a problem, and if so, tell me about it." The patients who act as though everyone is making a big deal out of nothing are the toughest to deal with, because they see no need for a doctor, a program, treatment, or making any changes in their otherwise perfect world. Besides, why go to all that work and self-sacrifice for nothing? They might ask us, "Why can't you all just leave me alone?" Their situation is like that of the alcoholic, which according to Alcoholics Anonymous is going to go on unchanged until they "hit rock bottom." Afterwards comes the admission that they have a problem, and they are unable to fix it on their own. At that point, recovery can begin.

If the patient is aware of her condition and its consequences, the next question to ask is whether she is willing to do whatever it takes to break free and get healthy again. How they answer this question will also provide a useful measurement to determine how well they will respond to treatment. The best prognosis will be when a patient knows she has a problem and is ready to get well.

Finding, Making, or Falling Into Space

Many times families have been split apart by someone's ED. The patient can become reclusive, difficult to deal with, and, if enabled by another family member, she can make the home life a living hell for everyone else. Although the best environment for healing includes the love and support of a healthy family, in more rare situations the patient is better off if, for a while, she detaches from her family and severs ties with them until she can get well. In any case, she will need to avoid the environments in which her ED developed and grew. If afterwards she is well enough to return home without relapse, she can rejoin her family on the condition that everyone works at improving their communication and the way they treat each other. So long as the patient is strong enough internally, she will be better prepared to deal with the unhealthy people in her life.

ED patients who go to college prior to treatment and discover their own space, may find that their condition is worsened. On the other hand, it may go into spontaneous remission. For some, living outside the close scrutiny of their parents makes it easier to surrender to unhealthy behaviors. Others, however, find a new personal freedom apart from the negative environment of their home and the unwanted and unpleasant attitude and actions of their parents. Returning home for the holidays will then become their challenge. Otherwise, detachment can sometimes become a win-win situation if both the parents and child feel relief during a period of separation, because the conflict, depression, and misery can dissolve with distance.

Obviously a healthy home that offers a supportive and loving environment improves the chances of a patient's recovery. Whatever the parents can do to build up and enhance the child's self-esteem will go a long way in her healing. In fact, if every parent would work at instilling positive self-esteem and self-confidence in their children, it could save a lot of young women from ever stepping into the dark world of EDs. Patients need to know their value to others and, hopefully, will become fully convinced that their self-worth is not based on superficial or external qualities like their appearance and that their bodies do not define who they are.

A healthy inner, spiritual life can be a tremendous asset in the battle with ED. When humans connect with the mystery of the universe, they become enlightened to its beauty, a beauty that they find in every person, and that the ED patient needs also to find in herself. To see our beauty as beings made in God's image is difficult for many people to accept, but when it is another stage in an ongoing spiritual journey, we learn to embrace it as part of our formation. Moreover, they must learn to find happiness from within and not just from without.

Radical Treatment Option

ED patients have come to my office weighing as little as sixty or seventy pounds, some being full grown, adult women. Some of them were already experiencing organ failure, broken bones, skin lesions, and other painful conditions. These women needed a higher level of care than my office staff and I could provide. For this reason, it is vital that the front desk has at hand a list of care facilities, treatment centers, and clinics that not only take ED patients, but also have a decent track record in sustained recovery. (There are too many clinics that will take a patient until her insurance dries up and then release her in a condition not much better than when she arrived.) There are excellent resources in which trained professionals provide the monitored care that the most desperate situations require.

After leaving the inpatient facility, I can follow up with the patient, track her progress, and make adjustments in her treatment as she gradually improves. Most patients, however, do not need hospitalization and can be safely and effectively treated in an outpatient setting. With the aggressive approach that is advocated by outpatient professionals, the patients will find at their fingertips all they need in order to recover.

For patients who are already ill or on the edge of serious physical breakdowns, due to malnutrition, monitoring is necessary in order to keep them supplied with phosphorous, magnesium, potassium, and other electrolytes. If a patient's metabolism has been compromised, then their bodies may not be able to ingest, assimilate, or derive any value from food. What happens when a woman's body is ravaged from poor nutrition is that her intestines may not be able to handle a sudden change in diet resulting in constipation, cramping, bloating, and other gastrointestinal problems. In such cases, she will require intravenous feeding until her digestive tract normalizes and her intestines can adapt to normal foods. Other patients may have developed an extremely rapid metabolism and require an elevated caloric intake to make even small gains in their weight. The meals, as well as monitoring their vital statistics, can best be done in an inpatient care facility, until she is stable enough to be in an outpatient environment.

The Team Approach

The most effective treatment for ED's is the team approach, which enlists the services of a psychologist (preferably one that has experience in and interest in the treatment of ED), a nutritionist (with the same qualifications), and a doctor who handles the medical aspects. Properly treating these patients will almost always require the application of medications, which we will soon discuss. A psychiatric consult can be helpful if the primary care doctor does not feel comfortable with medication management or if the case is more complex and the doctor is not available or trained in talk therapy. However, primary care doctors are in the ideal position to provide the most cutting-edge care to the most patients. The idea of the team approach is to address all aspects of these disorders by those who are best qualified to speak on each separate issue while working cooperatively for the improved health of the patient.

The Role of an Advocate

It may be helpful if one of the team members is a Recovered ED patient who knows the disorder from the inside out. This person can become the patient's advocate, because she too understands both the disorder and the patient in a way that goes beyond that of any other professional. Usually the advocate and patient will establish a special connection that softens the patient to whatever treatment is called for, no matter how rigorous. No one is more likely to get through to the patient than someone who has been in her shoes, has known her situation—even if not the same exact circumstances—seen the devil at the end of the road, turned around, recovered, and has lived to tell about it. Not only is the advocate a whole person today, but she is a model of what the patient can become and an example of how her life can be of value to other girls like herself.

The Role of the Psychologist or Psychiatrist

The psychologist works at uncovering the hidden circumstances that created and exacerbated the condition. They serve to prevent patients and their families from "sweeping problems under the rug," as we often do. Their job is to get at the serious childhood and adolescent issues that have yet to be resolved and dispel the illusions that have been left in the patient's mind as a result of negative programming through abuse or neglect. A psychologist or psychiatrist can also be invaluable in helping the patient understand her self-perception and why the way she sees her body image is distorted and untrue. The ongoing service of the counselor will include the important role of teaching the patient coping skills to enable her to deal with her former negative feelings, urges, and her current stressors.

The Role of the (Healthy) Family

Getting the family involved with treatment is very important, and the psychologist may recommend family sessions, in addition to individual sessions, with the patient. Parents often discover that they have desperately needed psychotherapy and/

or medications themselves, and that their mistreatment of their child was a carryover from the way they were treated as a child. If other family members receive therapy, not only will the home life likely get better, but the parent and child will share an understanding of each other's situation, and have a vocabulary to discuss their challenges, successes, failures, and ongoing journey.

Treatment of one person has on many occasions led to positive changes in the entire family. Open discussion about the subject has interested other family members in mood disorders and motivated them to get an evaluation of their own condition. For this, and a host of other reasons, it is important for all the family members to be involved in the treatment.

Even with the team approach it can be difficult to treat these patients optimally while family conflicts continue to flare up or family members continue to berate or tease the ED patient. To serve her best interests, every relationship that is important to the patient must be analyzed and corrected (or temporarily removed) if it is dysfunctional or in any way damaging to her self-esteem, increases self-destructive habits, increases irrational thinking and behaviors, or slows progress. Optimal progress includes a lot of healing of relations between the patient, parents and siblings.

Nutritionist's Role

A nutritionist initially gets involved to help stabilize the patient in a program that is based on a proper diet. Once the patient is in recovery, the nutritionist teaches her what a healthy diet is really all about—some junk food is required. The whole approach to consumption requires education, wisdom, and diligence over time.

Nutritional decisions for ED patients can be left to the nutritionist whose knowledge and training in the subject exceeds that of most medical doctors. Nevertheless, the doctor remains involved by tracking the patient's health and making certain she is following the nutritionist's instructions. Also, if the nutritionist has recommended any exotic supplements, the doctor needs to know about them and their possible interactions with prescribed medications.

Fear of Fat

Cutting fat out of their diet is perhaps the most common dietary behavior of anorexic patients. There are many other ways they can deprive themselves of nutrition, to be sure, but fat is definitely conceived to be an enemy. Patients can even become phobic and develop a fear of fats and any food they perceive as fatty and, therefore unhealthy, in their opinion. This would include extreme restriction of carbohydrates to decrease the glucose available to the body, that it could store as fat and, at the same time, try to stick to a protein-exclusive diet to increase their muscle mass. They may think that eating even small amounts of foods that contain fat and carbohydrates will then make them fat. That is simply not true though, as is discovered later when it may be too late.

Here we are face to face with one of the tragedies of ED's: the circumference of the ED patient's life becomes more and more narrow as time goes on and the disease progresses. Rather than eating foods they had previously enjoyed, or trying new foods, they often resort to eating "safe" foods, and this list can get quite short. Some of them eat the exact same thing every day and it is not uncommon for them to develop a lot of food rituals. (There are only so many ways you can eat a bland and static diet.) They tend to pick at their food and not eat anything they think will cause them to put on weight.

Fats are the most common "fear foods" and the foods ED patients are most reluctant to reintroduce into their diet. A good education regarding fats is absolutely necessary and the nutritionist will explain the importance of a balanced diet. A lack of fat in a person's diet can actually inhibit the development of lean muscle mass and other tissues. Instead, muscle wasting occurs when the body is deprived of all the nutrition it needs from a variety of sources. Rather than break into fat cells, if the body senses deprivation it will go first to muscle tissue for energy and save the fat in case the deprivation continues. In other words, those who eliminate fat intake from their diets actually make the fat they have more resistant to being burned up, because their bodies will stubbornly hang on to it.

Good and Bad Fats

The nutritionist will gradually introduce new foods into the patient's diet while working to dispel her unfounded fears. The nutritionist explains the difference between "good" and "bad" fats and the importance of balancing the right amount of protein, carbohydrates (bread, pasta, potatoes, rice, alcohol, sweets), and simple carbohydrates such as fruits and vegetables. The human body requires a good mix of basic foods and those foods must supply an adequate caloric content. Helping the patient take baby steps with regard to nutritional change is the nutritionist's job. In fact, if the patient were to regain her weight too rapidly, she may suffer both psychologically and medically. Rapid or excessive weight gain is a clue to the nutritionist that the reintroduction of a regular and healthy diet is moving too quickly. Rapid weight gain can result in refeeding syndrome which leads to edema, electrolyte imbalances, and possible cardiac problems and malfunctions in other organs.

The Doctor's Role

The primary care doctor plays a key role in assessing and treating EDs. Doctors are capable of making all of the important medical, psychological, and nutritional evaluations of the patient. The more times we take on these challenges, the better we become in diagnosing and treating them.

One of the doctor's roles is to explain the best treatment options available and observe the patient's decisions and course of action. The doctor also determines which ancillary health care providers may be necessary to enlist to pursue optimal treatment. They can also recruit the other team members and introduce them into the program as their services are required. The doctor also determines what lab tests are needed in order to evaluate the patient's overall condition and most pressing needs.

With the help of the psychologist and nutritionist, the doctor will try to draw the patient's focus away from weight and toward the goal of excellent health and becoming strong in mind and body. Many times we have to remind ourselves that treating these patients is a marathon and not a sprint. Therefore, we have to be patient and understanding while resisting frustration and the urge to give up on our patients. If the patient is medically stable, there is no reason to rush things. In fact, the paradox of rushing treatment is that it can backfire and cause an unnecessary delay in the patient's healing.

The importance of the role of medications cannot be overemphasized. These patients need aggressive medical management given the severity of their conditions and the risks that can occur with inadequate treatment. If an underlying mood disorder is contributing to their condition, or if their malnutrition has affected their thinking process, then the prescription of mood normalizing medications can greatly enhance their treatment and healing. They should be the rule rather than the exception.

The doctor needs to evaluate the risk factors in each ED patient's case to get them the appropriate care as quickly as possible and prevent them from doing permanent damage to their bodies or brains. The physician can also help the patient by walking through each part of her life, making certain that every important issue is adequately addressed and treated.

There is a reason why the work of a physician is referred to as a practice, and it is because we don't get it right the first time. Our knowledge is not static, and our experience is constantly expanding and deepening. Part of our practice involves trying new things to learn how to provide patients with the most effective treatment.

In order to treat patients well, provide the best health care, and be a source of constant reassurance, doctors need to be:

- Eager to constantly learn new information in every field of medicine, human behavior, and the interaction of the mind and body;

- Open to the insights, research, and experience of others;

- Humble;
- Genuinely interested in people as individuals and willing to take on the challenge of getting interested in those really difficult patients;
- Willing to try new approaches to the practice of treating patients with both medicine and personal interaction (e.g., "bedside manner").

THE LIMITATIONS OF "PURE REASON"

Medicine is a science, as is biology, physiology, cardiology, endocrinology, and all of the other "ologies" that represent all of the systems and structures of the human body and their functions. Therefore, the majority of a physician's training is in the sciences and every doctor to some degree, must be a scientist and think as a scientist. In fact, the scientific method that defines the nature, scope, and advance of medicine is exactly what I advocate in this book regarding chemical imbalances and mood normalizing medications.

There is a danger in getting so immersed in the reasoning and methodologies of science that doctors fail to see that their education is doing little good when they are dealing with an impaired mind. We may have bullet-proof arguments when we set out to convince the patient that she has a disorder and it needs to be corrected immediately, only to see her turn a deaf ear. Our logic may be infallible when we point out the damage she is doing to herself, but if her mind has already been busy justifying irrational behavior on the basis of personal needs for acceptance or safety, our reasoned warnings will sound weak and hollow to her. Keep in mind that many of these women have found some kind of security or protection for their wounded souls within their ED, so what they hear you asking of them is for them to take a huge risk— something that has never worked well for them—a walk across the tight wire without a safety net, a return to the emotional pain of a deeply scarred ego, and a supreme sacrifice. Reasonable or not, do not expect to have much luck chipping away at that granite mountain with your chisel of reason.

Most often, the ED patient's family, friends, and coworkers are at as great a loss as the doctor in trying to get through to her. Because they have not lived in her shoes, they have no idea what she has been going through internally and cannot comprehend her mental state. We might do well to note that a team of highly-trained and experienced physicians, psychologists, nutritionists, spiritual advisors, athletic trainers, and hospital clinicians, all working together have great difficulty in the recovery of ED patients. Of those who do not drop out, but stay with the program, the relapse rate is lower. Even the most loving families, working with friends who have the best intentions, are simply not equipped to take on the challenge of the patient's recovery on their own.

To put the central problem in the most clear language: As long as parents, doctors and others attempt to use rational thinking to win over an irrational mind, their efforts are doomed to fail. However, if the doctor as a scientist cannot use reason to convince a patient of her need for treatment, what option is left? The good news is there is hope and effective treatment options available.

First, the doctor needs to talk with the most rational family member. Additionally, the family needs to understand the limitations of logic when they get into arguments with their daughter. In fact, many arguments and shouting matches—along with the emotional misery they generate—can be diminished if the parent realizes the disorder may be preventing the patient from viewing the situation rationally. If the parent can take this big step, then they are ready for the next, and that involves making a sincere effort to understand how the patient thinks. If they realize the anguish she is trying to overcome and her desperate need to hang on to this coping mechanism then they will be drawn towards more compassionate, and therefore more effective, ways of interacting with her. A psychologist who is familiar with the mind of the ED patient and/or an advocate who has been there can be an invaluable resource to the family who seeks that greater understanding of the person they love.

TOTALLY IRRATIONAL?

Unless a woman's brain cells have significantly deteriorated through deprivation, or she was not mentally stable to begin with, she is not completely irrational. In fact, she usually demonstrates excellent logical skills in other areas of her life. One of my strategies in educating the ED patient is to point out that there are two parts to her mind, the rational part and the irrational part. Her rational mind is most important and more prominent, but it has to compete against the smaller, irrational part of the mind. Even though it is smaller, her irrational mind is louder, more demanding, and boasts greater promises that the rational mind and, so, usually wins whatever argument is going on between them. The irrational mind has a strong connection to emotions and feelings, so it is often used to justify fulfilling strong desires even if we know those desires to be wrong. In this and many other ways, the irrational mind drives her irrational behaviors.

I realize that when I am saying these things to the ED patient I may be wasting my breath. What I am attempting to do though is provide her with a new paradigm for understanding her current thinking and behavior. In other words, before I try to address her thinking, I try to get her to think about her way of thinking. I will also use what she recognizes to be logical in one situation and use an appropriate analogy to help her see how it can apply to her situation. If she resists with a counter argument, even if it is unreasonable, I acknowledge her point and affirm her as a thinking person. The worst thing that I could do at that moment is dismiss what she says or in any way trivialize or minimize her as a person. To reject her argument out of hand would be to crush her soul once again.

If the patient will acknowledge that she understands what I mean by a rational and irrational mind, and if she can see how the dominance of the irrational mind in any particular area will impair sound judgment, then I suggest that she will continue to run into the same walls and roadblocks again and again if she keeps going down the same path. If she is willing to explore her current state of misery, I can show her that it is the result of repeated behavior and that it is time for a change—that is, if she is interested in experiencing happiness. I encourage her to take a turn in a new direction, and I promise to walk with her and assist her if she is willing to do so. No doubt the turning is easier said than done, but at the outset all we are looking for is the slightest indication that she is willing to take a chance with us. Hopefully, we will earn her trust, develop a rapport, and walk them into treatment with the seriousness her condition deserves.

In summary, if a doctor is unable to reason with an ED patient—or is limited to working with a smaller base of reason and a greater depth of personal concern—other options include:

- Try to create new paradigms through which the patient can understand herself, her condition, and her thinking about her condition.

- Seek to build a rapport with ED patients.

- Tell the patient compelling stories (a good story is not without logic, but it tends to be hidden more than in an argument. The power of storytelling is emotional and, therefore, has a greater likelihood of success with irrational patients whose emotions are exactly what they perceive to be in jeopardy).

A FEW OTHER GENERAL GUIDELINES WOULD INCLUDE:

- Expect resistance. Even when patients are rational enough to concede your point of view, they will usually continue to resist until they have hit bottom. There have been times when, at precisely the right moment, I have convincingly told a patient, "There's no door out of this room you have locked yourself in. You need to try a different key in a different lock. It is time to make a change in your thinking and behavior." Then the patient responded with something like, "Yeah, I know you're right and I'll probably do what you say, but not until I lose five more pounds." In other words, she has not been truly convinced that her program is not working and will not work. I do my best to convince her otherwise.

- Use the patient's fear of weight gain as a loose measurement of her distortion of thought. I may ask her what her "ideal" weight would be, and record this information for future reference. An indicator like this is not meant to be precise, but rather to serve as a benchmark for treatment by indicating how distorted her body image is.

- Do not go over the patient's changes in weight from one appointment to the next—that is, unless you intend to use it strategically to keep her motivated. Instead, steer the conversation in a different and positive direction. Help her to think about other things in the world besides her body.

- Ask the patient to keep a chart of how often she looks at herself in a mirror and to write down on the chart what she sees. Sometimes the simple act of writing, which engages other areas of the brain than speaking, can help to open their eyes to the truth. At the least, you or the psychologist can use this information in a cognitive behavioral approach to train her to evaluate flaws in her own thinking and change her mind.

- Provide her with a professional assessment of her body image. Remember when doing this to be firm, but fair.

- Be generous with forgiveness and patience for both the patient and family. Also, ask that they be patient with you, and understand that although physicians are agents of God for healing, they are not God himself, not infallible, and cannot work miracles.

Classifying Eating Disorders

We want to find categories which match the neurological patterns, personal behaviors and symptoms of ED. Finding the right classifications will direct us in the proven ways of effectively treating the condition. At this point in my practice I have found it useful to relate ED's to a subtype of obsessive-compulsive disorder (OCD). Obsession describes the thinking pattern in regard to their relation to food, nutrition, weight, and, in the case of bulimics, purging. Compulsive manifests itself in frenetic (i.e., exercise), addictive, ritual or repeated behaviors. We are actually scratching the surface here regarding the total range of parallels between these two disorders, but this is enough for now to help us understand why the medications that are used to effectively treat OCD have also proven useful in the treatment of ED's.

There have been a number of my ED patients who truly wanted to give up their behavioral patterns, but found it almost impossible because of their underlying obsessive thinking. These are also patients who would be at high risk for relapse unless their obsessive tendencies were addressed and reduced. Mood normalizing medications have been applied to ED patients with OCD (or similar symptoms) with dramatic results. Some of these patients have progressed so far that they tell me they never knew happiness until they began taking medications in conjunction with treatments for their ED. The same results are reported by ED patients who manifest other sorts of neurochemical imbalances.

However, I must add that ED patients are more difficult to deal with and help than the typical OCD patient. OCD may be very responsive only to a stand alone serotonin reuptake inhibitor at high dosages. ED patients, on the other hand, will likely need augmentation through combining medications to achieve the same level of improvement, with the goal being full remission. Medications serve to reduce obsessive thinking and anxiety, allowing her enough space, energy, will, and presence of mind to change her behaviors. They are better equipped to stop binging on too many "comfort foods" because a chemical imbalance that had them feeling needy and desperate for comfort has been corrected. ED patients derive enormous help from mood normalizing medications that relieve them of anxiety and depression, bipolar disorder, and other conditions that result in stress to the body. Moreover, these medications enable them to control stress. To attempt recovery from an ED without medications is like trying to push a huge boulder up a steep hill. You might succeed, but you are more likely to be crushed by your failed attempt.

Specific Uses of Medications

Given the importance of mood normalizing meds in the treatment of eating disorders, what is the best approach to administering these medications? The answer is actually the most cutting-edge treatment for ED's: The off-label use of medications, which we will come to momentarily.

For Anorexia Nervosa

Recommended medications to start with:

- Selective serotonin reuptake inhibitors such as Prozac (fluoxetine), Zoloft (sertraline), Lexapro (escitalopram), Paxil (paroxetine), Celexa (citalopram), Luvox (fluvoxamine) or a "super SSRI" such as Viibryd (vilazodone) or Trintellix (vortioxetine), usually at low to medium doses.

- SNRIs may be better for some, especially if somatic symptoms and anxiety are predominant.

- Atypicals for more difficult-to-treat patients, which are not uncommon.

- Lamictal (lamotrigine), Deplin (L-methylfolate) and others more rarely.

For Bulimia Nervosa

Recommended medications to start with:

- Selective serotonin reuptake inhibitors such as Prozac, Zoloft, Lexapro, Paxil, Celexa, Luvox, Viibryd or Trintellix, often at higher doses.

- SNRIs may be better for some, especially if there are coexisting somatic symptoms or high anxiety.

- Topamax (topiramate), Neurontin (gabapentin), and other "anti-seizure" medications can be very useful augmenting agents. Topamax is excellent for control of appetite (and the temptation to binge), with other potential benefits being weight loss, paincontrol, and anxiety control. Topamax helps control carbohydrate and sugar cravings, thus improving control of their decision-making.

- Atypicals for more difficult-to-treat patients.

Some patients will manifest a sensitivity to medications early on, which is another good reason to begin at a low dosage and gradually taper it upwards, as needed and as tolerated. In this way I am able to recognize those who show a special sensitivity to a particular medication and then decide whether to stay with it at the low dose, reduce the dosage even further, stop it, or shift to a different medication and see how the patient adapts. I treat patients who do not manifest sensitivity to their medications more aggressively. Achieving optimum benefit of medications as quickly as possible is quite an effective blow to the disorder. If the patient is forced to wait too long in order to experience some kind of benefit from her meds, she may more easily lose heart and give up. Medications are almost always needed and should not take long to work if they are prescribed in the right way. Attrition during treatment is probably the most common form of relapse, especially if not treated aggressively enough with medical, psychological and spiritual support.

Providing Comfort and Encouragement

These patients almost always require ongoing encouragement, comfort and affirmation. Many of them turned to their ED in an attempt to escape the barrage of negative comments that assaulted them in their homes. If the doctor acts authoritatively, like a parent, the patient will be less likely to follow the treatment plan. However, if they find in the doctor someone who cares for them, treats them with respect and compassion, and is there to help them, they will be more apt to follow instructions and do whatever is requested. If, in this way, the doctor can enlist the patient's will to change, healing is likely to follow, because the majority of these patients can do whatever they set their minds to do. (Remember that some of them have the will to starve themselves.)

Kindness and comfort will help these patients move past the initial anger and embarrassment that comes with being dragged to the doctor's office. Trust is a huge factor in every doctor-patient endeavor, and the patient with ED needs to know as well as any other patient that her doctor is sincerely on her side and wants only the best for her. For this reason, patients need to be allowed to say anything, divulge anything, question everything, and speak freely, so that they can form a partnership with the doctor in reaching their mutual goals. If these patients can be convinced to play an active role in their own treatment by working, not only with me, but also with their parents and other team members, they may not only get better physically and emotionally, but one day they will be able to pay it forward and help rescue another ED patient. This is the proof of their soul's healing and the next goal beyond their own full recovery.

The Long, Winding, and Rewarding Road Home

Even with the very best treatment approach, the actual process of getting better is long and frustrating, not only for the patient, but for the family, doctor, and everyone else involved. Some patients respond slowly and others do not respond at all in spite of aggressive treatment, hospitalization, outpatient trials, and the ongoing love and support of their family. Eating disorders are very serious conditions and need to be treated with the concern that we give to any life-threatening illness. Early detection and treatment gives a young woman the best chance of recovery, but an ounce of prevention is always better than a pound of cure.

Frustrating though it may be, there is no greater feeling of gratification or reward than to make this journey with a patient and see her in full remission. Eating disorders are as fascinating for their complex mix of physical and psychological factors as they are difficult to treat. Once you learn enough about the ED's stranglehold on its victim, you learn to appreciate any improvement, even if it does not occur as favorably or as quickly as we might wish. The patients and families are always grateful for even the slightest motion upward, out of the dark pit and into the light. They are also forever grateful to the doctor who stays the course and helps them fight the battle.

Eating Disorder Summary

Anorexia Nervosa Warning Signs:

1. Loss of menses (menstrual cycle) or irregular menses
2. Strange eating behaviors i.e. food rituals
3. Preoccupation with foods (such as obsessiveness regarding cooking, nutrition, caloric content and other obsessive details about food).

(Vegetarians are at higher risk)

4. Rapid weight loss
5. Denial of hunger
6. Claiming to look and feel "fat" when the reality is different (what I refer to as distorted body image or body dysmorphism)
7. Decreased stamina with regard to physical and mental activities
8. Frequently feeling cold
9. Thinning of hair
10. Dryness and thinning of skin
11. Negative mood changes
12. Weighing oneself frequently
13. Excessive exercise
14. Obsessively dieting when not overweight
15. Under-eating coinciding with negative mood changes
16. A higher potential for abusing stimulants, whether by prescription amphetamines, OTC products with caffeine and other natural stimulants, "power drinks," cocaine, methamphetamines and other forms of "speed."

Warning Signs of Bulimia Nervosa:

1. Binging followed by dieting, followed by binging, etc.
2. Overeating and purging coinciding with negative mood changes
3. Purging in various ways: Vomiting, laxative use, diuretic use, over-exercising

4. Excessive use of energy/diet pills and supplements
5. A higher potential for abusing other types of amphetamines, i.e., cocaine, crystal meth and speed in whichever form
6. Binging on sugars, carbs and other high-caloric foods
7. Leaving for the bathroom right after meals
8. Secretive binging by one's self and secret purging (this occurs more in the evening)
9. Feeling "lack of control" regarding eating habits
10. Planning ahead opportunities to binge and purge
11. Judging oneself based on weight

There are other warning signs of bulimia nervosa, which overlap with the symptoms and signs of anorexia nervosa and other ED's. By now, though, we are not at all surprised, because overlap has been one of the recurring themes in our study of chemical imbalances and mood disorders. In fact, the more precisely we can identify and target specific problems when there is a multiple diagnosis, the better our strategy for treatment.

Medical Complications of ED:

1. Abnormal menses (irregular or absent periods)
2. Dry, cold, thinning skin
3. Feeling cold frequently
4. Slowness of thought

5. Erosion of gums and teeth
6. Hemorrhoids
7. Constipation
8. Acid reflux/heartburn
9. "Irritable bowel syndrome" (bloating, cramping, pain)
10. Stunted childhood and adolescent growth
11. Increased risk of osteopenia and osteoporosis at a much earlier than average age
12. Abnormal liver enzymes, which reflect the strain on the liver and, at times, the need to metabolize itself when there is an inadequate nutritional supply otherwise
13. Electrolyte abnormalities, i.e.: sodium, potassium, calcium, carbon dioxide, etc.
14. Increased risk of edema resulting in body swelling in various areas (legs, arms, abdomen, face, etc.)
15. A low white blood cell count hints towards "fat malnutrition," with a lowered immune system and an increased risk of infection
16. Anemia which can be due to inadequate intake of iron, B12, folic acid or others, due to lack of proper nutrients
17. Dehydration with resultant complications
18. Decreased estrogen, testosterone and other hormones
19. Thyroid abnormalities (What appears as low thyroid on lab results may actually be due to malnutrition)
20. Cholesterol abnormalities (lower numbers than average, or the opposite. It depends on the liver.)

21. Blood pressure abnormalities (usually low)
22. Kidney abnormalities
23. Pancreas abnormalities
24. Gallbladder abnormalities
25. Shrinkage of brain and other tissues that the body depends on
26. Heart rhythm abnormalities
27. Increased risk of heart attacks
28. Increased risks of strokes
29. Increased risk of sudden death

HEALING
— THE —
MIND AND BODY
VOLUME 1
SECOND EDITION

— SECTION V —
CONCLUSION

THE ART OF MEDICINE

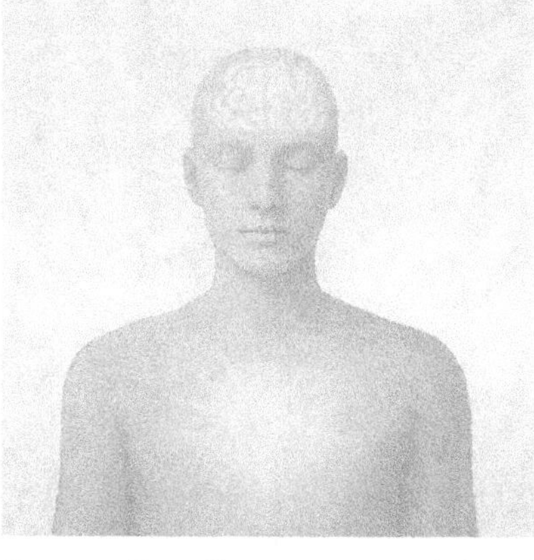

PAUL D. CORONA, M.D.

Chapter Thirteen

The Art of Medicine

In the previous chapter I said that science is foundational for the practice of medicine. To fully appreciate the doctor's profession as a calling rather than a job, we need to think of medicine as an art as well as a science. Growth, development, and progress in any field requires a mixture of creativity and knowledge. This dynamic mix of traditional wisdom and educated innovation is necessary at this stage of clinical history in the diagnosis and treatment of mood disorders.

During the nineteenth century there was an unfortunate rupture between science and art, the philosopher and the poet, reason and faith. Prior to that time, the advance of science had to be taken forward by people who could reason as a scientist, but create like an artist. Inventors of technology had to be, in a word, inventive. Something happened, though, in the worldview of western civilization that polarized science and art. As a result of this fracture, scientists were perceived as hardheaded bean counters driven by logic and abhorrent of anything frivolous, and artists were perceived as lazy dreamers who could barely function in the real world. The premises and objectives of science and art seemed to conflict with each other—science being the life of the mind in developing medicines and technologies to improve conditions for the survival of the human species, and art being the life of the soul to give meaning to the survival of the human species.

Conflict is an unfortunate paradigm for understanding the relationship of science and art. Perhaps a better word is *tension* because it acknowledges the real differences between the two disciplines, yet defines them in a complementary rather than oppositional way. Ever since Einstein, no physicist has been embarrassed about also being an artist or even being a person of faith. The tension between art and science may represent a divided house, but it is still one house and each benefits from its relationship to the other. Science has not only given artists new technologies (e.g., egg based paints, followed by oil-based paints, followed by acrylic-based paints), but its integration of the artists' creation helps to maintain the integrity of art. Art, on the other hand, reminds scientists to revere life and not merely dissect and classify it. Art serves to inject passion and creativity into science and to push it toward humanitarian ends by recreating scenes of human drama or natural beauty that jog our memory. The why questions in life are as important as the what and how questions.

To put this as succinctly as possible, the combination of science and art yields the results of the scientific method in the promotion of goodness, truth and beauty.

So, taking our cue from Einstein, who said, "The only real valuable thing is intuition," I would argue that the doctor's educated intuition is what defines the art of medicine. Nowhere in the entire field of medicine is the exercise of intuition revealed more than in the diagnoses and treatment of malfunctions in the human body and mind. Intuition, though, does not mean doctors pull cures out of thin air or spend their day following hunches. Rather, intuition is a sense of knowing something without going through all the stages, steps, and proofs to reach a conclusion. Experts in every field are able to make quick decisions in problem solving because they are informed by experience, can eliminate many dead-ends without having to examine each one, and they have a mental check list that they may not even know about, yet have tweaked and abbreviated through the years, and arranged in a sequence from most likely problem to least likely.

For example, a doctor in residency and straight out of med school will listen to a patient's complaints, take an inventory of the patient's symptoms, and then begin to eliminate the possible conditions that could cause those symptoms one by one, precisely by the book, until the condition is diagnosed and the correct course of treatment is determined. The whole process could take hours or even days. A veteran doctor with years of experience can see the same patient and in five minutes prescribe medication and send the patient home. If asked how he was able to intuit the diagnosis so quickly, the expert doctor may not even know the mental processes that led to the quick decision. However, what may look like paranormal insight or a lucky guess to the casual observer, is actually the brain selectively accessing its complete store of knowledge, along with multiple associations with familiar situations from the past, and a few important pieces of information. This is educated intuition in action, and after a few years of working with patients, doctors need to trust that instinct.

The Art of Medicine in Action

Artists train themselves, either naturally or by much practice, to be observant, therefore they tend to notice what others miss. In medicine, this not only requires looking at visible symptoms, damaged tissue, and lab reports, but carefully listening to the patients. Listening is both general and selective. This is because information will be crucial to the art form. Some will be interesting, especially in getting to know the person. However, some will be irrelevant. Therefore, in my practice, I am paying particular attention to how the patient's thoughts, behaviors, medical problems, and neurochemicals all interrelate and whether there is harmony or an obvious breakdown in one or more of these relationships. The successful composition that I seek to produce is a healthy human being and hopefully a changed life. The joy of my art often comes to me in the exam room when the patients report the good news of how much better they are feeling and functioning when their chemistry is balanced. To be honest, I did not hold out much hope for some of these people when they first entered my office.

I have found that no patient is totally hopeless. If we cannot achieve full remission, we can certainly achieve marked improvement. We can take out our brushes, applying highlights to create a more complete and beautiful work. When we do see the masterpiece of full remission, I continue to add touch-ups with the assistance of the patient so that by working together we can improve my patient's mental and physical health and perhaps take it to an even higher level.

Finding Satisfaction

My father, who has developed real estate for a living, stood one day before a completed project and said to me, "God help me, I love it so." Money may define the professional, but passion defines the artist. How fortunate it is for those of us who are able to make a living at doing what we believe in and love. I have seen truck drivers tie complicated knots in less than ten seconds, yet with a choreographed grace and smoothness that revealed a genuine commitment to, and investment in, their work. Approach any profession with passion and you will become an artist.

> *Do you see a man skilled in his work?*
> *He will serve before kings;*
> *He will not serve before obscure men.*[1]

Like an artist who steps back from his canvas, or reads her poem in print, or sells that first novel and savors the moment of a completed work, I get an overwhelming feeling of satisfaction when my patients return to normal life with an appreciative smile.

The Medium of Medical Artistry

Some people may think of medication and technology as the medium of medical art, but these are merely tools like the poet's typewriter or the painter's brushes and paints. The blank canvas of medicine is the human person who is a composite body, mind, emotions, and spirit. Like other artists, the doctor's first step is the careful study of the subject to be drawn, the story that needs to be told, the theme that needs to be explored, or the melody that needs to be played. Then, once I determine what my subject demands, I begin to apply my tools, using intuition and creativity to add color, form, and shading, to bring forth the beauty that lies within the

1 Proverbs 22:29, The New International Version of the Bible.

person. My goal: a changed life, and when I am doing my job correctly, that is what I see.

I do not take a dehumanizing view of my patients, treat them as if they were a blank sheet of paper that needed my scribbling, or think of them as a block of marble that I must sculpture. Far from it! Rather I see them for who they are, the men, women and children who think and hope and dream just as I do, and who are far more complex than the most elaborately designed and equipped computer. They are strong yet fragile, lost yet moving forward, lonely yet defensive, needy yet skeptical. Each of their life-stories are award winning if anyone would take the time to listen. I want to know each of my patients, know them as persons and help to heal them as such. That is why the art of medicine is the most challenging of all forms of art and why the doctor must use intuition and not just reason, because humans do not always live, function, and suffer according to logical rules.

A big difference between conventional art and the art of healing a human is that the former is not prone to change over time while the latter cannot help but change. Once a painting leaves the gallery or a musical piece is played before a live audience or released in an album, the artist does not have to deal with it again. The figures on the canvas are not going to move, nor will the notes on the music sheet. The human body and brain, however, are constantly evolving and changing, which requires a lifetime of artistic additions and alterations.

I do not accept patients making excuses for their symptoms, such as, “I'm just getting old” or “Of course I feel miserable, just look at my life. It's a mess!” Quality and enjoyment of life is not age related or dependent on pleasant circumstances—otherwise, no one would be happy, ever! Whether we enjoy life depends on what we put into it, where we find contentment, and the relationships we build with others. We need the presence of mind to be able to keep going into life every day. In recent years I have devoted my whole heart and soul toward assisting patients into a healthier presence of mind.

Maintaining Improvement

Throughout this book I have stressed the complex interplay of mind and body at every level. To heal one, we must address and mend the other. Thoughts, both negative and positive, affect feelings and moods, moods affect health, health affects thoughts and moods, tension creates painful knots in various muscle groups, pain causes stress and anxiety, and so on and so on. The conditions and problems that arise when the balance of chemicals affects a malfunction between the nervous system and the rest of the body are at the heart of a health crisis that amounts to an epidemic, although most people are not even aware that such a thing exists. If they are made aware of the crisis and its magnitude, they do not know there is a solution at hand.

At present, we do not have any tests that indicate how much serotonin is being released in the brain or whether it is moving forward from one neuron to another as it should (much less having any means of testing the condition of a person's soul). We only have the patients, their symptoms, their stories and our intuition. Therefore, doctors must take enough time with each patient to ask them how they are feeling and what they are feeling, paying close attention not only to what they say, but how they express themselves when they speak. Many people, especially elderly women and almost all men, even more so those who have fought in a war, tend to downplay and hide symptoms from doctors, telling them only what they want the physician to know. However, if we become skilled listeners, we will be able to discern when they have not told us everything. Rather than sigh with frustration, we must tell ourselves, "Alright, Mr. Holmes, the game is afoot! Let's begin our investigation into the truth."

In the examination room, doctors need to remind themselves, "Before me there is a beautiful work of art. The problem is that it has been vandalized, worn down over time, its colors are faded, and its canvas is torn. Now what do I have to do to restore this work to its original glory?" If we stop, relax, and breathe we will do a better job of solving the case. Or, to switch metaphors, we have a job before us like that of Indiana Jones when his father was dying and he had to choose the right chalice to save his father's life. Getting to the chalice, the Holy Grail, the Cup of

Christ, though requires finding solutions for complicated puzzles. That is where we stand, between the sick and their cure. We must solve the complicated puzzles in order to achieve the coveted prize and optimal treasure of mind-body health.

Every time I see a person suffering with fatigue, insomnia, pain, depression, anxiety, or any other persistent physical or mental symptoms, something within compels me to do everything in my power to make a difference in their lives. Once we turn the corner toward relief and healing, I ask them to let me know if they feel they have begun to slip back into the old feelings. I stay with them to get them back on track. For these patients, what is at stake is their life. For that reason, their health care is a lifelong process. All of my training, experience, instincts, and skills converge in the exam room where I sit with my patient and together we make life changing decisions.

Claiming What's Ours

Can we agree that nothing less than full remission should be the standard of health care? How can a doctor settle for slight improvement, or even significant improvement, in a patient's condition if full remission is possible? If we set a higher standard for the medical community—and there is a lot of room for improvement—we will see a lot less suffering for individuals, their families, their communities, and our whole society.

Can we agree that patients and doctors are the most critical decision-makers regarding the patient's health care and treatment? We need to guarantee their freedom to decide between available options without interference from government, insurance companies, pharmaceutical companies, the American Medical Association, or anyone else. I pray for the day when there are no formularies, authorization requests, drug overrides, patients having to choose an HMO versus a PPO, or any of the absurdities that are wasting our time and money, or compromising our emotional and physical health, while becoming more and more of an emotional drag on everyone.

Can we agree that patients are the ultimate victims in our twisted system and their health is being compromised by institutions whose concern for money or power override any possible interest in people? Can we agree that this system needs to be changed? On behalf of suffering human beings, doctors need to be able to prescribe medications and other forms of therapy without being questioned and second-guessed by those who know very little about human wholeness. For example, pharmacists routinely try to convince patients to settle for a knock-off medication because it will cost the insurance company less money while increasing profits for the pharmacy. (There is a higher markup, and thus more profit for the pharmacies, if they can convince patients to accept generic medications.) Has it occurred to anyone that this great fraud is perpetrated by sheer greed, because insurance companies are among the wealthiest corporations in the world?

Can we agree that doctors need to regain the passion they had when they chose a career in medicine? Since that time, the mountains of paperwork, the bribing of insurance companies, the loss of income through revisions in the health-care system, and the growing demands of government, have quenched the fire in many doctors. No wonder so many of them have become cynical and decided that, like everyone else on the ladder above them, they had better watch out for themselves and try to make as much money as possible, giving less and less attention to the emotional needs of their patients. Do we really want to be treated by physicians who are burnt out by the onerous system that casts its dark shadow over their profession?

Regardless of all the troubles, grievances, and abuses of health care today:

- I am excited about the future of medicine and the emerging role that neurochemistry and mood normalizing medications will play in our daily practices and in our lives.

- I am excited about the ever increasing body of knowledge we are acquiring regarding the mind-body connection and how that plays out in health care. For someone who enjoys learning, I cannot imagine a more exciting field to follow.

- I am excited about seeing people improve: people who others have given up on, people who never thought they would get well, and people who would have been lost if someone had not told them about the importance of the chemical balance in their brains and nervous systems. I can guarantee that the more physicians get comfortable treating the mind and body, the more excited they too become about the balance of one's neurochemicals because of the results they will personally witness.

- I am excited about the possibility of newer and better medications becoming available in the future (but do not disregard the value of today's medications). As new medications are developed in labs, the focus will be on increasing effectiveness and minimizing side effects. I can also imagine a day off in the future—hopefully not too far off—when sophisticated technology will be able to determine what is happening in a human brain, what neurochemicals are malfunctioning and for what reasons, where the brain needs the most attention and how to service it, and perhaps using our growing knowledge of genetics to solve problems, such as Parkinson's Disease, Alzheimer's Disease, Autism, and other disorders that may currently not be recognized as being related to imbalances in one's neurochemistry.

- I am excited about the dramatic changes in a person's life when he or she returns to the office to tell me, "I can't believe how much better I feel." Even then, if they have not reached full remission, I tell them I am happy that they feel better, but I also explain that our work is not done until they feel their best.

WOW

The most important thing to know about the Wonder of Optimal Well-being, is that anyone can benefit from it, and if you are not as happy as you have ever been in your life, that lost joy can be returned to you. If people think of you as a crank, and you do not know why you are so grouchy all the time, you can begin testing with your doctor to see if it may be a mood disorder. If you are depressed, hopeless, or if you ever entertain the thought of suicide, I urge you to act on your newfound knowledge and seek treatment. My sincere hope is that, if you do not know the WOW in your own life, you will discover it sooner rather than later. Do not let your mind grow accustomed to these negative feelings or think that you have to learn to live with them. I can assure you that you do not. Regardless of how hopeless you feel now, I promise you life can get much better. You simply cannot imagine what happiness awaits you.

Your life can be reconfigured from the inside out, opening up doors to the simple pleasures hidden in every moment, allowing you to feel at home in your body, and giving you a positive outlook on your life. In full remission, you will look back at your former self and wonder how you could have ever felt that low, that dark and hopeless. If you have kept a journal, you will go back and read it as if someone else much less fortunate than you had written on those pages. You will be a different person, and you will enjoy the new you.

The art of medicine, as it applies to you and I, and anyone else with whom you share this information, can be summed up in a well-known statement: "Perfection is impossible to achieve. However, if we strive for perfection we may be able to achieve excellence." We will achieve excellence, and that has been my goal for you and your family. Perfect or not, lets take the next steps to bring to completion the masterpiece that you are in mind and body.

Dr. Paul

ACKNOWLEDGMENTS

There are so many people I want to thank that I hardly know where to begin, so please bear with me. I would like to thank Carol Cada, who has handled all of the dictation of the original draft as well as the multiple rewritings of this and the next book. She has spent countless hours trying to keep up with my frenetic pace, and I appreciate her time, effort, and input.

I would like to thank my editor, my pastor, my mentor and my good friend, Chuck Smith, Jr. He has taken what I originally wrote and helped bring the book to life. He has helped to teach me how to write and how to communicate more effectively, and I will always be grateful for his help when it was so needed.

I would also like to thank my editor extraordinaire, Tom Herron. He has been such a pleasure to work with, and I look forward to working with him on many future projects. I have learned a lot about writing through the arduous editing process, and he has been a great teacher throughout this experience. Writing is a collaborative process, and I have appreciated my editors during this journey. More recently, thank you to Lisa Burnett for her final editing of the second edition of these first three books.

I have had an incredible book team to work with. I especially want to thank Viki Mason, who has handled the typesetting and layout of the first edition. Thanks, Viki, for your tireless efforts during this arduous process.

More recently, special thanks to Karen Corriente, who handled the design and layout of the second edition of my first three books, as well as my newest three. She has spent countless hours dedicated to helping me. Thank you, Karen.

Thanks to Christi Koop for the original cover designs and illustrations in the books, and more recently, thank you to Jaime Simon, who did such a good job designing the new covers of my first three books.

Special thanks to my awesome assistant Leslie Perez whom I spend every day with in my office. She is such a pleasure to work with. I also want to recognize my previous assistant, Fabiola Baltazar.

I would also like to thank all of my patients over the years who have been so supportive and encouraging. They have been my greatest teachers, since I have learned to do what I do by listening attentively to them and working closely with them towards our mutual goal of optimal mind-body health.

I want to recognize my alma mater, the University of Southern California. My wife and I are big fans of their football team, and we are hoping that Lincoln Riley, as well as his coaches and team, will take us to new heights. Fight On Trojans! I also want to mention my other favorite team, the Nebraska Cornhuskers. Go Big Red!

Some of my best teachers and mentors have been my favorite authors who have personally inspired me, and we obviously share a passion for writing. These authors include Ayn Rand, C.S. Lewis, Terry Brooks, Terry Goodkind, Robin Hobb, Tad Williams, Anne Rice, Jim Butcher, Brandon Sanderson, Suzanne Collin's, J. K. Rowling, Joe Abercrombie, J. R. R. Tolkien, Dan Brown, John Green and Gillian Flynn. I have especially enjoyed the Shannara series by Terry Brooks, and my favorite childhood books were *The Chronicles of Narnia* by C.S. Lewis.

I would like to also mention some recent books I have read that have had a real impact on me. Malcolm Gladwell's *The Tipping Point* has helped me to understand how ideas affect social changes of epidemic proportions, and his book *Blink* gave me personal insight as to how and why I think and act the way I do. Dr. Martha Stout's book *The Sociopath Next Door* is certainly disturbing but also certainly very compelling and impactful, and I think it's important for everyone to read this in order to protect themselves.

My all-time favorite book is *Atlas Shrugged* by Ayn Rand. I encourage all to read it, as well as all of her books, since doing so necessarily changes how you look at and understand the world so much more clearly. Her philosophy of Objectivism has helped to clarify my political and moral thinking with regard to not only Medicine but life in general. She brilliantly explains why individual rights and Capitalism are the only moral forms of government, and her dream, as well as mine, is that this great country again finds its moral compass in order to be a truly free and great nation. Her intellectual heir, Dr. Leonard Peikoff's article entitled "Medicine, The Death of a Profession," was very influential early in my career by explaining how and why Medicine has gone wrong and what we can do to fix it.

Last but not least, I want to thank my wife, Denise, my son, Logan, and my daughter, Baylee. I want to thank my father, Arthur, who has been immeasurably supportive of me over the years. Special mention to my cat Seymour, the best cat I have ever had, along with our dog JG. They bring so much joy to our lives. I hope you enjoyed reading this book.

www.ingramcontent.com/pod-product-compliance
Lightning Source LLC
LaVergne TN
LVHW052023200926
848481LV00005B/1567